# Which Tests For My Unborn Baby?

## A guide to prenatal diagnosis

Lachlan de Crespigny
with Rhonda Dredge

OXFORD

Melbourne
Oxford   Auckland   New York

OXFORD UNIVERSITY PRESS AUSTRALIA

Oxford   New York   Toronto
Delhi   Bombay   Calcutta   Madras   Karachi
Petaling Jaya   Singapore   Hong Kong   Tokyo
Nairobi   Dar es Salaam   Cape Town
Melbourne   Auckland

and associated companies in
Berlin   Ibadan

OXFORD is a trade mark of Oxford University Press

National Library of Australia
Cataloguing-in-Publication data:

de Crespigny, Lachlan James Champion.
    Which tests for my unborn baby?

    Includes index.
    ISBN 0 19 553094 2.

    1. Prenatal diagnosis — Popular works. I. Dredge, Rhonda.
    II. Title.

618 32075

Edited by Sarah Brenan
Designed by Sandra Nobes
Illustrations by Juli Kent
Typeset by Abb-typesetting Pty Ltd, Collingwood, Victoria
Printed by Impact Printing Victoria Pty Ltd
Published by Oxford University Press,
253 Normanby Road, South Melbourne, Australia.

Cover photograph and Figure 1.1 are from *A Colour Atlas of Life Before
Birth — Normal Fetal Development*, by Marjorie A. England, Wolfe Medical
Publications Ltd, London, 1983.

# CONTENTS

# ACKNOWLEDGEMENTS

I am indebted to my many colleagues and friends who have read part of all of this book. They offered their critical comments and each contributed expertise in their own way. I especially wish to thank Dr Eric Haan for his work in Chapter 5 and elsewhere, plus Dr John Hobbins, Dr Hugh Robinson, Dr George Kossoff and Professor Roger Pepperell; and finally my parents, Jim and Joan.

I also wish to thank Ms Julie Kent-Corston who prepared the diagram and Mr Robert Madden at the Royal Women's Hospital, Melbourne for assistance with the photographs, Miss Margaret Cooke who prepared the graph for figure 5.4, the cytogenetic department at the Royal Women's Hospital for the two karyograms and Dr Marjorie England and Wolfe Publications for allowing me to use the anatomical pictures on the cover and in figure 1.1. I am grateful to Ms Lou Sweetland from Oxford University Press without whose enthusiasm this book would not have begun, and Sarah Brenan for her skilled editorial work. I particularly wish to acknowledge Mrs Kerrie Carson for her tireless work in typing this book.

L. C.

I wish to thank the Murdoch Institute for Research into Birth Defects, and Ann Robertson at the Royal Women's Hospital for their expert guidance on genetic counselling. Paramount, though, is my appreciation of the many women who willingly shared their experiences of prenatal diagnosis.

R. D.

*Science has promised us truth . . . it has never promised us either peace or happiness*   (LeBon)

*I can promise to be sincere but not to be impartial*   (Goethe)

*Life is the art of drawing sufficient conclusions from insufficient premises*   (Samuel Butler II)

*Most ignorance is vincible ignorance — we don't know because we don't want to know*   (Aldous Huxley)

*Everybody wants to be somebody, nobody wants to grow*   (Goethe)

# INTRODUCTION

Testing a baby before birth for genetic or growth abnormalities is a young and rapidly changing field of medicine. Until twenty years ago, women had no choice but to accept the risks dealt out by nature of giving birth to a malformed baby. Without intervention, this occurs in about 4 per cent of births, an incidence high enough to cause major parental and medical concern.

The first revolution in prenatal diagnosis was the application of ultrasound to obstetrics, making it possible to visualize the developing baby. Techniques for analyzing the amniotic fluid surrounding the baby followed. For the first time, parents could find out in advance about certain serious abnormalities such as neural tube defects, Down syndrome and some severe brain deformities and metabolic disorders. They could then decide whether or not to continue the pregnancy. More recently, a method of sampling the developing placenta has allowed earlier diagnosis and sophisticated techniques such as DNA analysis have led to the detection of an ever-increasing range of disorders.

But like anything that deals with matters of life and death, these tests raise some agonizing ethical dilemmas. Despite the scientific advances of testing, intervention usually provides only one choice: termination of the pregnancy or not. There are no cures for most of the major malformations. Most parents believe that children with Down syndrome or spina bifida have such a reduced quality of life that they decide to terminate a pregnancy if given this diagnosis. The decision is more difficult, however, with some other abnormalities. Babies born with sex chromosome variations may be virtually normal, or they may grow up with a mild mental deficiency. Testing has just become available for Huntington's chorea, an inherited gene disorder of the nervous system that is debilitating in later life. Among the many dilemmas raised by this advance is the question of the ethics of terminanting a life that may be normal and productive until the age of 40 or beyond. A medical geneticist, commenting on a meeting where a method was presented for prenatally identifying another gene disorder — osteogenesis imperfecta — expressed her view on the new technology. As a person afflicted by this fragile bone condition, she knew it intimately. 'The scientist announced this was a disease no child should be allowed to bear. I felt discriminated against and glad that I was not conceived in the biotechnology era. Every life contains some suffering but I think mine has been useful.' Other issues raised by testing include its impact on the whole experience of being a parent. In her well-publicized book *The Tentative Pregnancy*, Barbara Katz Rothman examines the idea that testing interferes with maternal attachment to the developing baby.

While society grapples with the increasingly complex questions raised by the new techniques, individual women and couples are forced to make their own particular decisions. It is for these people that this book is written. Our major concern is the issue of informed consent. How much information is provided to women before they decide to go ahead with the procedures? Are they aware of the risks and limitations of the tests or what is involved if a result leads to a decision to abort a baby at 20 weeks?

Many women agree to testing without a clear idea of what it involves or what they will do in the case of an abnormal result. They have just discovered they are pregnant, may have no knowledge of Down syndrome and other abnormalities, yet they are asked to make a decision about whether to have an invasive test and which one. As one genetic counsellor puts it, 'I don't think it's appreciated just how distressed women can become when faced with these decisions. There is an enormous paucity of information about prenatal testing'.

It is the aim of this book to fill in those knowledge gaps; to describe the advances in prenatal diagnosis while making clear what it cannot do. The new tests do not magically prevent birth defects. It is estimated, for example, that one in 200 newborn infants are severely retarded. Chromosome abnormalities, the major reason for testing, account for only about 40 per cent of these. There are many other disorders, some environmental, some genetic, that no currently available test can diagnose.

At their best, however, the tests can be life-saving. Ultrasound can forewarn of the existence of several rare conditions that require urgent medical attention at birth. The genetic tests are also extremely useful for women at higher risk of carrying a child with certain birth defects. The chances of a woman conceiving a child with a chromosomal disorder begin to rise at 30 years of age and escalate rapidly after 35. There are also those with a family history of genetic disease who may run a risk as high as one in two of passing it on to their children. For these people, prenatal testing can mean the difference between an average family life and one of heartbreak. Many such couples would choose to remain childless if testing was unavailable.

In every pregnancy there are reasons for special concern. The following statements are particularly common: 'I am worried about this baby because it is my first'; 'I am getting old, so I need to take special care of this pregnancy'; 'I drank too much in early pregnancy. I hope my baby is OK'. People are also more aware of fetal abnormalities — affected children are no longer hidden away and we are more likely to come into contact with them. Many mothers' concerns focus on whether the baby is normal rather than on miscarriage or premature labour, both of which are more common than an abnormality.

This fear of carrying a malformed baby, coupled with an increasing tendency for women to put off child-bearing to a later age, has meant an escalating demand for prenatal testing. The use of ultrasound is now routine in many countries and most couples in high-risk groups choose to have one of the more invasive tests. Acceptance is as high as 80 per cent within these groups in Western Europe, the United States and Australia. In some countries, there is a trend to allow women to have prenatal diagnosis at a younger age. Some see danger in this approach, as exerting indirect pressure on women to accept testing and further medicalizing the pregnancy experience. The trend towards widespread prenatal diagnosis is likely to escalate, however, as a new system of screening is offered to all pregnant women to detect those at higher risk of Down syndrome. This method, which is based on testing the mother's blood, is outlined in Chapter 9.

There are undoubted, albeit small, risks of miscarriage associated with the invasive tests which usually rely on sampling amniotic fluid or cells from the developing placenta. For this reason, doctors would not recommend they be routine procedures in all pregnancies. The perception of those risks also varies according to the personal history of the woman contemplating testing: if she has already had several miscarriages, a stillborn child, a sudden infant death or a long period of infertility, any risk may be seen as threatening.

This book aims to provide a factual account of the range of procedures available to pregnant women. Remember that, as in any skilled field, the expertise of operators performing ultrasound and genetic tests varies. Results and risks quoted in this book assume that state-of-the-art equipment is used by experienced and skilled operators. We will suggest guidelines to help you assess whether you are gaining maximum care and safety.

You may not wish to read this book from cover to cover, but select the relevant chapters. If you are less than 35 years old and have had no previous baby with spina bifida or chromosomal abnormalities, Chapters 1–4, those on ultrasound, will be most relevant. If you are over 35, read the chapters on amniocentesis and chorionic villus sampling as well. A number of commonly asked questions are answered at the end of the relevant chapter.

If you are having trouble deciding whether testing is right for you, the experiences of others outlined in Chapter 8 may help. You should discuss any specific concerns with your doctor and if you wish for further information, ask to be referred to a geneticist. These are doctors who specialize in birth defects, their genetic component and the effects of any drugs or infections during pregnancy.

# 1 NORMAL EARLY DEVELOPMENT OF YOUR BABY

One of the most satisfying things about performing an ultrasound examination, is observing the pleasure couples gain from seeing their baby on the screen. Most are stunned that it is so human-like, as early as 10 weeks. 'Look it's moving already.' 'I can see its arms.' 'Is its heart already beating?' These are typical of the kind of comments an ultrasound operator will hear every day. They are also indicative of the general lack of knowledge within the community about early fetal development. Most people are surprised at just how quickly their baby develops from a single cell. Before covering the technique of ultrasound in depth, therefore, we will describe the baby's development and relate this to what you will see on the ultrasound screen.

## Time of Conception

On average, conception occurs around 14 days after the first day of your last menstrual period, i.e. in the middle of the next cycle. While most women know the date their last menstrual period began, very few can be *certain* when they conceived unless they were having special investigations as part of treatment for infertility. In obstetrics it is therefore not possible to use the real date of commencement of pregnancy and for convenience the pregnancy is said to begin on the first day of the last menstrual period.

# Early Development

It is extraordinary just how quickly your baby develops. It changes from a single cell two weeks after your last period began to having a very human appearance eight weeks later. A baby has fully formed arms, legs, face, head and body at 11 weeks after the last menstrual period began (see figure 1.1). From 11 weeks until delivery is a time of growth and maturation, most of the baby's basic structures already being fully formed (see table 1.1).

From a medical viewpoint, knowing the timing of your baby's development is important in assessing the possible impact of teratogens. This is a general term for substances such as Thalidomide or viruses such as rubella (German measles) which can damage the unborn baby, during a particular period of its development. Babies who develop an abnormality of the upper arms or legs due to Thalidomide, for example, must have been exposed to the drug when these were developing between 5 and 9 weeks. Similarly, a baby with spina bifida, a condition in which the spinal canal does not fully close, shows defective development prior to 6 weeks when the spine is forming.

## Movements

Pregnant women are amazed to see their baby moving on ultrasound at 8 to 9 weeks as they are unable to feel the movements until around 18 to 20 weeks, or sometimes a little earlier in second and subsequent pregnancies. The mother will only start to feel movements when the baby is strong enough to kick hard against her abdominal wall. Even after the onset of movements (quickening) only a small proportion of them are felt. When ultrasound shows a vigorously moving baby late in pregnancy, you still may feel nothing, and may not do so for many days. This situation is actually a blessing for the mother — to be aware of each movement from 8 weeks until delivery would be exhausting.

# The Placenta

The pregnancy becomes attached to the wall of the uterus on day 20, six days after fertilization. Once attached, the very early pla-

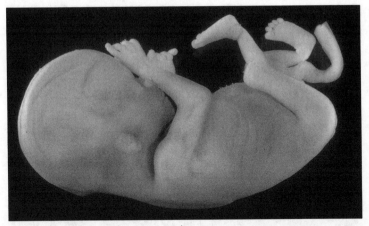

Fig 1.1 A normal baby at 10–11 weeks.

centa — the chorion — starts to function to provide oxygen and nutrients to the baby and to remove wastes. If the placenta separates from the uterine wall at this stage, the baby does not have any way of receiving oxygen and nutrients from the mother, so it dies immediately.

Until 8 weeks the chorion appears on the ultrasound screen as a thick white layer totally surrounding the baby (see figure 1.2). In the early weeks of pregnancy you therefore cannot tell where the placenta will develop. At nine weeks the chorion begins to thicken in one area while thinning elsewhere. By 10 weeks it is clearly seen on one wall of the uterus (see figure 1.3) and is now called the placenta rather than the chorion. Both the chorion and placenta are made up of cells derived from your baby. It is these that are tested in chorionic villus sampling (CVS).

The early placenta has enormous reserves and powers of regeneration. Even if it becomes partially separated from the uterine wall by blood clot it can recover and a healthy baby result. Even late in pregnancy there is enough reserve for the baby to survive even if half or more of the placenta separates.

The exchange across the placenta occurs without any mixing of the mother's and baby's blood (see figure 1.4). They are totally separated by a thin membrane although at times small amounts of the baby's blood can cross into the mother's circulation. (In the

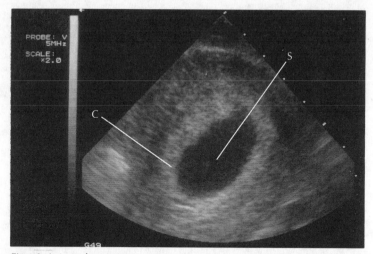

Fig 1.2 A 6 week pregnancy sac (S). The chorion (C) surrounds the pregnancy sac and appears as a white rim, the dots on the right of the picture are centimetres.

Fig 1.3 A 10 week pregnancy showing the head (H) and body (B) of the baby surrounded by the fluid in the pregnancy sac (S). The chorion (C) is now thickened in one area where the placenta will develop.

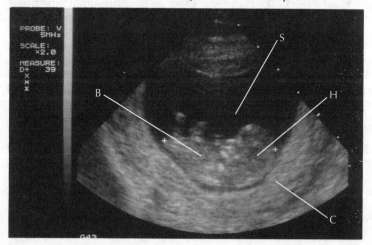

same way, non-identical twins with a single placenta have separate circulations, each using its own half of the placenta independently. Identical twins, however, usually do have some communication between their circulations.)

At any stage of pregnancy it is not important how the placenta looks on ultrasound but rather how well it functions. Many babies have died with a placenta that looks absolutely normal. Ways of testing its function include looking at the growth of the baby, its well-being and the amount of amniotic fluid present. The texture of the placenta itself is usually immaterial.

# ▌ Growth

Most mothers are anxious to find out if their babies are growing normally, particularly if a previous baby was especially large or

Fig 1.4 As this diagram of the placenta shows, the mother's and baby's blood does not mix, but exchange of nutrition and waste occurs across the villi. Blood from the baby's cord passes through villi which are surrounded by mother's blood in cavities called sinusoids.

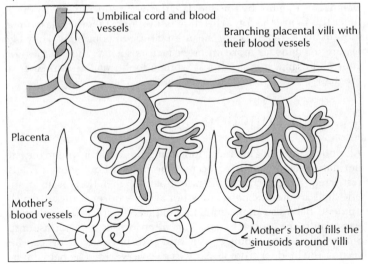

Umbilical cord and blood vessels

Branching placental villi with their blood vessels

Placenta

Mother's blood vessels

Mother's blood fills the sinusoids around villi

small, if there has been a complication such as bleeding, or if they feel or look small compared to others at a similar stage. In fact, in the first half of pregnancy, all babies grow at much the same rate. Measuring parts of the baby such as its overall length or head size can therefore reliably show the degree of advancement of the pregnancy. If growth falls behind the expected rate prior to 20 weeks it may mean dire consequences for the baby, but these circumstances are rare.

Table 1.2 summarizes the sequential development of your baby and indicates its approximate length, weight and the amount of amniotic fluid present. Until 20 to 24 weeks pregnancy, all babies grow at the same rate. Therefore the measurements in the table will closely reflect those of your own baby. After 24 weeks however, there is an increasing discrepancy between big and small babies, so the table will not necessarily closely reflect the measurements of your own baby. There is also a wide range in amniotic fluid volume throughout pregnancy, the volumes presented in the table being averages.

The large differences seen in the sizes of babies at birth come mostly in the second half of pregnancy, particularly the last few months. You can see from the chart that at 28 weeks an average weight is 1.1 kg but by the due date the average is more than three times this figure (3.4 kg). This shows how important these last three months are in determining the ultimate size of your baby. How big *you* are depends far more on other factors such as the tightness of your abdominal muscles (most women look smallest in their first pregnancy), and your own body build.

# ▋ Organ Function

All your baby's organs must function from early in pregnancy if normal development is to occur. The baby whose movement is restricted (as can occur in the rare situation when there is no amniotic fluid around the baby) may not achieve normal muscle development. Babies swallow amniotic fluid (see figure 1.5) which then passes into the stomach. This can often be seen on ultrasound. Similarly, kidneys produce urine and with ultrasound this can be seen in the bladder from as early as twelve weeks. The baby inter-

TABLE 1.1    MAJOR EVENTS IN PREGNANCY

| **Gestation** (weeks) | **Milestone** |
| --- | --- |
| 0 | 1st day last menstrual period |
| 2 | Release of egg (ovulation) |
| 4 | |
| 6 | |
| 8 | Movements begin |
| 10 | CVS performed |
| 12 | |
| 14 | |
| 16 | Amniocentesis performed |
| 18 | Ultrasound to check baby's development |
| 20 | Movements usually felt |
| 22 | |
| 24 | Babies delivered have a chance of survival |
| 26 | Babies delivered have a reasonable prospect of survival |
| 28 | |
| 30 | |
| 32 | |
| 34 | Babies delivered unlikely to have serious complications due to prematurity |
| 36 | |
| 38 | |
| 40 (9 months + 7 days) | due date |

mittently empties its bladder but rarely totally because it can nearly always be seen on ultrasound.

The baby even practises breathing motions prior to birth. While its oxygen exchange is across the placenta from your circulation, it does expand its chest intermittently, especially later in pregnancy. This aids lung development and prepares its chest muscles for breathing after birth. The passageways to the lungs are full of fluid which moves up and down with each 'breath'.

# ▌Amniotic Fluid

Once your baby's kidneys start functioning at 8 to 9 weeks they soon produce most of the amniotic fluid. This is then removed when the baby swallows and is absorbed in the intestine. The whole volume of amniotic fluid is turned over at least once per day. The amount increases very rapidly in early pregnancy. At 6 weeks there is approximately 1 ml, by 10 weeks 34 ml and by 16 weeks 200 ml. As shown in Table 1.2, this continues to increase slowly throughout the pregnancy until approximately 32 weeks and then decreases slightly until the due date.

There is a wide variation in the amount of fluid around babies at all stages of pregnancy. A little more or less than average in any particular pregnancy certainly does not suggest a problem. The baby needs very little fluid around it to allow normal development. Only if the fluid is very much increased or decreased would your obstetrician be concerned. The worry is usually not the altered amount of fluid itself but rather what has *caused* this to happen (see Chapter 2).

The content of the amniotic fluid tells us a great deal about the

Fig 1.5 Prior to birth babies swallow the fluid around them. In this profile view the baby's nose (N) lips (L) and chin (Ch) and chest (Cs) are visible. Note there is fluid (Fl) which appears black in the mouth and over the tongue (T).

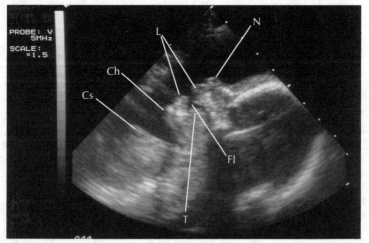

baby, since it contains cells from your baby. These are shed from the skin, lining of the airways, and other parts of the baby's body. Although most are dead, some are still alive and can be grown in the laboratory after the fluid is sampled at amniocentesis. It is then possible to determine the chromosome count of the baby, or look for hundreds of other genetic diseases.

There is much more than just baby's cells floating in the amniotic fluid. Many sorts of protein, salts and hormones are found in it. The levels of many of these can be tested to study specific functions of the baby. One example is alpha-fetoprotein (AFP), the level of which is raised in most babies with spina bifida. This will be discussed further in Chapter 5. A further example is a test for bilirubin level in the amniotic fluid which is used to assess the severity of blood group incompatibility in Rhesus disease. This will be discussed in Chapter 10.

# Questions

IS IT A BIG BABY?    The answer to this question will not be evident if the scan is carried out in the first half of pregnancy. Even if your baby is going to be much larger or smaller than average at birth, it is likely to be the same size as everybody else's at this stage.

IS THE PREGNANCY ATTACHED PROPERLY?    This concern is raised by mothers who have bleeding in early pregnancy. If the baby is alive, then the pregnancy is properly attached. It attaches to the wall of the uterus 6 days after you conceive, so that by the time you have seen it on the ultrasound screen it has been attached for some time.

DOES THE PLACENTA LOOK NORMAL?    Placentas are remarkably consistent in appearance on ultrasound, and in early pregnancy the texture almost always appears the same. Occasionally towards the end of pregnancy the placenta may show some calcification and other changes, but even these do not mean there will be any problem with your baby's growth or development. The important thing is the function of the placenta and this is assessed by looking at the amount of fluid around the baby, by the baby's growth or by other tests.

TABLE 1.2    MAIN STAGES IN BABY DEVELOPMENT

| Completed Weeks | DAYS | CROWN–RUMP LENGTH (cm) | CROWN–HEEL LENGTH (cm) | WEIGHT (Gm) |
|---|---|---|---|---|
| 0 | 0 | | | |
| 1 | 7 | | | |
| 2 | 14 | | | |
| 3 | 21 | | | |
| 4 | 28 | | | |
| 5 | 35 | | | |
| 6 | 42 | 0.3 | | |
| 7 | 49 | 1 | | |
| 8 | 56 | 1.6 | | |
| 9 | 63 | 2.4 | | |
| 10 | 70 | 3.3 | | |
| 11 | 77 | 4.3 | | |

| FEATURES PRESENT | APPEARANCE ON ULTRASOUND | VOLUME OF AMNIOTIC FLUID (ml) |
|---|---|---|
| First day of last menstrual period | | |
| Ovulation (release of egg from ovary) | | |
| Embryo implants in the wall of the uterus. | | |
| Eye and ear start to form, head and tail present. | Chorion becoming visible, pregnancy sac and baby not seen. | |
| Arms start to form. | Pregnancy sac visible but not the baby. | |
| Spinal canal closes around spinal cord. | Embryo and its heart movements visible. | 1 |
| Head and body well established. | Different structures of the baby cannot yet be made out. | 2 |
| First movements occur. Chorion still totally surrounds pregnancy sac. | Head can be differentiated from body. | 10 |
| Fingers separated but toes still united. Chorion thicker where placenta will develop. | Arms and legs can be seen. | 18 |
| Heart fully formed, mature placenta. Now called a fetus. Human appearance with eyes, eyelids and ears. | Starts to look human with face, arms and legs seen. | 34 |
| Bowel returns inside baby's abdomen. | Spine, skull and some internal organs visible. | 51 |

TABLE 1.2   CONTINUED

| Completed Weeks | DAYS | CROWN–RUMP LENGTH (cm) | CROWN–HEEL LENGTH (cm) | WEIGHT (Gm) |
|---|---|---|---|---|
| 12 | 84 | 5.5 | | |
| 13 | 91 | 6.8 | | |
| 16 | | | 15 | 0.1 |
| 20 | | | 23 | 0.4 |
| 24 | | | 28 | 0.6 |
| 28 | | | 37 | 1.1 |
| 32 | | | 43 | 1.7 |
| 36 | | | 47 | 2.6 |
| 40 | | | 49 | 3.4 |

* Crown–rump length: the length from the top of the head to the tip of the bottom.
† Crown–heel length: the length from the top of the head to the heel when baby is lying flat at its full length.

| FEATURES PRESENT | APPEARANCE ON ULTRASOUND | VOLUME OF AMNIOTIC FLUID (ml) |
|---|---|---|
| Urine production. Sex can be identified. | | 74 |
| End of first 3 months (first trimester). | Improving views of baby's structure | 110 |
| Occasional mothers feel movements | Usually can obtain good views of baby's organs. | 200 |
| Most mothers now feel movements. | 'Screening' ultrasound performed 18–20 weeks. | |
| Babies delivering after this time have a chance of survival. | Parents can still see good lifelike pictures of their baby. | |
| Eyelids open. Most babies delivering now will survive. | Baby larger than transducer so parents find pictures harder to interpret. | 1000 |
| Babies delivering now less likely to have severe complications of prematurity. | Most scans performed are to check baby's growth or the site of the placenta. | |
| Nails reach finger tips | | |
| The due date (9 months + 7 days after the first day of last menstrual period) | | 600 |

# 2 WHY HAVE AN ULTRASOUND SCAN?

Ultrasound examinations use sound waves above the range of human hearing to provide images of your baby. The advantages of being able to look at the baby before birth has made the technique an almost universal part of safe obstetrics in Western countries. It is currently the safest and most non-invasive method of checking on the development of your baby. With the increasing sophistication of equipment, ultrasound has also become an invaluable method for diagnosing pregnancy complications and many fetal abnormalities.

In this chapter we will examine some of the common reasons for having an ultrasound examination. One of life's great frustrations is the variation one will find in 'expert' opinion. This applies to obstetricians and their views on when to order a scan. Some believe that everyone should have an ultrasound examination, while others say that it is only necessary when specific complications are suspected. If you are interested in those views — ask your doctor. It is our hope that the information provided here will help you form your own opinions.

## Main Reasons for an Ultrasound

Increasingly doctors are suggesting that all pregnant women should have an ultrasound examination. The four main reasons are:
(i)    **Dates** It is impossible to be absolutely certain how far on a pregnancy is without an ultrasound examination. Confirmation or establishment by ultrasound of a due date simplifies the management of many obstetric complications.

(ii)   **Multiple pregnancy** Without ultrasound multiple pregnancies are usually diagnosed late in pregnancy, some twins only being detected after delivery of the first baby. This poses added risks to the babies.

(iii)  **Placental localization** A scan will pick out those who are at high risk of having a placenta which is too low in the uterus (placenta praevia). This can lead to bleeding late in pregnancy, in which case hospitalization is necessary.

(iv)   **Malformations** Many malformations can now be detected by ultrasound. The range is so wide that these are covered separately in Chapter 4 with a description of how they are visualized during the examination. Most babies with abnormalities are born to women who have had no previous problems. Therefore, if scans were restricted to those in high-risk groups, most abnormal babies would not be picked up before birth.

There is also another factor which should not be forgotten. Parents often find their ultrasound examination an enjoyable and emotional experience. Pictures of the baby are obtained which unquestionably help parents bond to their unborn child.

The other main reason for ordering an ultrasound is to assist in the diagnosis of pregnancy complications. This has simplified their management and allowed a more scientific explanation for the range of symptoms that can cause concern during pregnancy.

# ▌Arguments against Routine Ultrasound

There are several disadvantages in everybody having an ultrasound examination. One is the financial cost to both the individual and the community. Another possible drawback is ill effects from the ultrasound itself. As discussed in Chapter 3, it is now considered most unlikely that ultrasound used for diagnosis can cause damage to the baby.

Another argument occasionally put against ultrasound is that it may lead to unnecessary intervention in the pregnancy. This could arise where there was an incorrect diagnosis of a problem which led to inappropriate action. Such situations provide a strong argument for the use of good equipment and experienced operators, and if there is any doubt about a diagnosis, a second opinion; they do not constitute a valid argument against ultrasound itself.

There is no doubt that ultrasound can determine dates, and detect placental site, a multiple pregnancy and many fetal abnormalities. A recent large study has shown that ultrasound screening also reduces significantly the number of deaths immediately before and after births. The cost benefit of ultrasound is a complicated issue. To scan all women is costly, but it is also expensive from a public health standpoint to pay for the care of undiagnosed problems.

## Timing of the Scan

The appropriate timing for your ultrasound examination depends on the reason for having it. If it is undertaken because of bleeding, that dictates when it is carried out. If it is important that your dates be known exactly, then the scan should be done in the first few months of pregnancy. For most women, however, the best time to have a scan is at approximately 18 weeks. This is still quite a good time for checking the dates — to an accuracy of within one week — and multiple pregnancy and the placental site can be readily seen. At this time your doctor can usually also obtain excellent views of the structure of your baby so he or she will be able to pick up many abnormalities. Your obstetrician may have good reason for wanting to have the scan at a different time, but would discuss this with you.

## Checking your Dates

If the only thing that ultrasound could do was tell the age of a pregnancy it would still have a most important role to play in obstetrics. The management of complications is critically dependent on the age of the pregnancy. Before ultrasound, it was not possible for an obstetrician to be sure whether a small baby in late pregnancy was the result of incorrect dates or inadequate growth. A number of women were confined to hospital, often for many weeks, in an effort to resolve this question. Widespread use of ultrasound has solved the problem because the age of any baby can now be known precisely.

This also means of course that the exact time of conception can be known, which is important if the baby might have been exposed to some potentially dangerous substance in early pregnancy. As women do not know they are pregnant until after they miss a period, and occasionally much later than this, they may unwittingly expose their baby to various substances or medications. It then becomes important to know the date of conception to work out at what stage of the baby's development the exposure occurred. Another reason for wanting to know the exact date is if there is doubt about the paternity (father's identity). Knowing the exact date of conception may tell somebody who the father is.

No matter how sure you are of when you conceived, it is known that occasionally mistakes occur. Even though you know the date of your last period and even if you feel you know when you ovulated, nature can fool you. Occasionally what seems to be a 'last normal menstrual period' was in fact bleeding in early pregnancy. If you conceived a month earlier and had some vaginal bleeding of an amount and timing very similar to your period, then how would you know? The surer you are of your cycle and conception date the less likely it is that such confusion will occur, but it still occasionally happens. Also, many women do not ovulate exactly two weeks after the last menstrual period, which complicates the calculations of the due date.

Similarly, obstetric examination may not give a precise date. If, for example, you have a fibroid or ovarian cyst or even just a little urine in your bladder then the uterus can feel a lot bigger than it really is. Often there is no obvious reason why you feel big or small. Moreover, when an examination is done, the obstetrician feels the overall size of the uterus, which includes the placenta and amniotic fluid. The examination is made through your own body tissues so that if you are fatter or thinner than average, this may cause confusion.

None of this discussion means that everybody *must* have an ultrasound examination to work out how far on they are. If you are sure when your last period began and your obstetrician feels that your uterus is an appropriate size for these dates then there is only a low chance that these clinical methods will prove to be inaccurate.

Don't forget that ultrasound does not tell you when you will deliver your baby but rather when it is *due* to be delivered. You may deliver your baby well before the expected date or after it. There is no way with ultrasound or any other method of predicting when your labour will actually commence.

# ▌ TIMING OF SCAN FOR CHECKING DATES

The earlier the scan is performed the more accurate is the due date it will give you. This is because no matter what race the parents are, how big they are, or how big the baby is destined to be at birth, its growth rate is fixed in the first few months. At 7 to 10 weeks ultrasound will give a due date with an acuracy of a few days, and this is therefore the best time for determining the date of conception. Between 13 and 20 weeks the accuracy is to within one week either way. The nearer you get to your due date the less accurate it becomes. In the second half of pregnancy there is a large biological variation in growth rates, resulting in normal babies' birth weights being between about 2.9 kg and 4.0 kg. Since we work out the age of a pregnancy by measuring parts of the baby, clearly the method will be very inaccurate in the last few weeks of pregnancy. The date estimated then by ultrasound may be as much as three or four weeks out.

# ▌ MEASUREMENTS FOR DETERMINING DUE DATES

Until 13 weeks the measurement taken is the 'crown-rump length' of the baby (figure 1.3). This is a measurement taken from the top of the baby's head to the tip of its bottom. If the baby is too small for such details to be seen then the baby's longest measurable length is taken to be the crown-rump length.

After 13 weeks any number of different measurements can be taken. Most people would measure three or even more parts of the baby to help get the most accurate due date. The first used and probably still the most accurate measurement is that of the head —

the biparietal diameter (BPD). The BPD is the largest measurement taken from one side of the skull to the other. While this can vary somewhat with the shape of the baby's head it remains the most widely used measurement.

The second measurement is that of a long bone in one of the baby's limbs, usually the femur (the bone of the thigh — see figure 4.8). The size of the baby's abdomen is usually also measured, particularly late in pregnancy. While the abdominal size is a most important measurement in assessing the growth of your baby (which we will look at later in this chapter) it can also be used to help determine how far on you are. Any number of other measurements can also be taken, but if the due dates provided by these first measurements correspond there is little to be gained.

# Multiple Pregnancies

Approximately one in 80 pregnancies conceived without the aid of medical treatment are twins and 1 in 6400 triplets. Ultrasound can identify the number of babies present from very early on in the pregnancy. No matter how early you are scanned, it is unlikely that ultrasound will miss twins. As a scan provides a section all the way through the pregnancy, the babies cannot 'hide behind one another', so avoiding detection.

It is not until about 6 weeks that the babies and their heartbeats become visible in each of the pregnancy sacs. At this time, the number of babies seen is likely to be the number that you take home. If one dies, it will stay inside your uterus until the time of delivery, unlike a single pregnancy which eventually miscarries after the death of the baby. Its presence should not affect the growth and development of the other baby. Without ultrasound, a pregnant woman would not be able to tell that a twin had died: the other baby usually keeps growing normally, the placenta still operates and there is no bleeding.

## IDENTICAL TWINS

Approximately 70 per cent of twins are non-identical (dizygous — coming from two separate eggs fertilized by two different sperm)

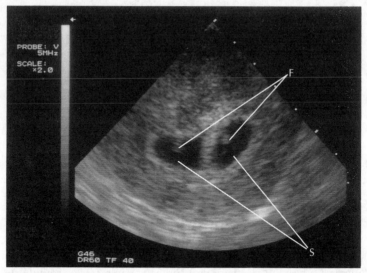

Fig 2.1 Twins at 6 weeks (S=sac, F=fetus). There is a thick line separating the fetuses, indicating they are likely to be dizygous (from two separate eggs).

and 30 per cent identical (monozygous — from one egg which separates into two very early in development). Ultrasound can usually indicate whether your babies are likely to be identical. In the rare case where they are both in the same pregnancy sac without any membrane between, then they are always identical. If they are in sacs separated by a thin membrane, they are also likely to be identical. A thick membrane usually indicates they will not be identical (figure 2.1). The presence of a single placenta, however, does *not* tell you whether the babies will be identical. Approximately half of non-identical twins share a single placenta, although they each have their own circulation through separate parts of the placenta. Identical twins usually, however, have some mixing of their circulations at the placenta.

# ▌ SIAMESE TWINS

Siamese or conjoined twins are very rare — approximately 1 in 50 000 live births or 1 in 600 twin pregnancies. Nearly all twins are in their own separate sacs which makes it impossible for them to be joined. Once the membrane between your babies has been identified then the possibility of joined twins can be immediately excluded.

# ▋ EXTRA SCANS

It is more difficult for your obstetrician to feel each baby individually through your abdominal wall if you have a multiple pregnancy. It may be suggested, therefore, that you have an ultrasound examination in the last few months of pregnancy to check the growth of each baby. If it is difficult to feel which way the babies are lying, then this may be checked as well. There is no general consensus as to if and when such scans should be carried out.

# ▋ Complications in Pregnancy

# ▋ BLEEDING IN EARLY PREGNANCY

Bleeding in the first half of pregnancy is called a threatened abortion. If you are going to miscarry this is almost always the first sign you will have. About one in seven recognized pregnancies miscarry. In some pregnancies, however, women have bleeding even though the baby is healthy and growing normally.

Ultrasound is the only test which will tell you if the baby is alive in early pregnancy. A pregnancy test only tells you that you are pregnant, and you probably already know that. Pregnancy tests merely tell you that there is some placental tissue present, they give very little information about the well-being of the baby itself.

Some obstetricians would always order an ultrasound examination if there is bleeding in early pregnancy . They would argue that if the baby has died further bleeding is likely to continue until some action is taken, therefore the earlier the ultrasound examination is carried out, the better. Other obstetricians, on the other hand, might feel that if the uterus appears on examination to be an appropriate size for your dates and the bleeding has not been heavy there is a high chance that your baby will remain healthy and that it would be a waste of time and resources to perform a scan. Neither viewpoint will be correct in every case. Ultrasound does provide a good indication of whether you will miscarry. If the baby is alive, with its heartbeat visible, there is approximately an 85 per cent chance that it will continue to develop normally.

It is worth noting that if bleeding occurs either the baby has already died and you will miscarry, or it will continue to develop, with little increased chance of having an abnormality. The blood that is lost is your own and not the baby's. The placenta has great powers of recovery, so even if there is clot in the uterus it does not appear to cause any damage to the baby's health or growth.

# ▌ MISCARRIAGE

It may surprise you to know that if you miscarry the baby nearly always has died some weeks or months before, usually in the first 8 weeks of pregnancy. The miscarriage itself may occur as late as 20 weeks. In the meantime you still feel pregnant, as the placenta continues to function and produce pregnancy hormones. You may even feel that you are still growing.

If your obstetrician does an internal examination, he or she may notice that your uterus feels a little smaller than it should be but otherwise there is no way of telling that the baby has died. Often the symptoms you notice in early pregnancy, such as nausea, start to lessen after the baby's death but these are often improving at this time anyway so are difficult to interpret. Don't be surprised and disappointed in your obstetrician if you do have a miscarriage and find on the scan that the baby has been dead for some time and nobody has suspected it.

If the baby grows for at least the first 6 weeks and then fails to develop it can usually be seen on ultrasound and is called a 'missed abortion'. This is not 'missed' because it is lost but rather because it has died and your body has not yet expelled it (i.e. there has been no miscarriage). If, on the other hand, the baby died earlier than this then it will be too small to be seen on ultrasound and it is called a 'blighted ovum' (i.e. a pregnancy without a visible fetus — see figure 2.2). In either case, if nothing is done after your baby has died then you will ultimately miscarry. As this may take many weeks or months, and may be associated with heavy blood loss, most women and their obstetricians believe that it is much better and safer to curette the uterus. Either situation will have no bearing on future

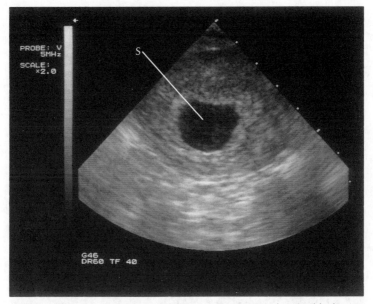

Fig 2.2 A blighted ovum: this pregnancy sac (S) contained no visible fetus. It may have been present earlier but died when it was so small it could not be seen with ultrasound.

pregnancies — after one miscarriage, the risk of a miscarriage in the next pregnancy is not increased.

If your pregnancy is 6 weeks or less when you have the scan performed, your baby's heartbeat cannot yet be seen. It is of course impossible to know whether it cannot be seen because it is too early or because the fetus is dead. Even if you believe you are further on than the size of the pregnancy suggests, it is hard to be certain, so it is best to repeat the scan one week later. Depending on the experience of your doctor and whether or not he has a vaginal scanner, it is sometimes even much later than this before he can give you a definite answer on ultrasound.

If your baby is alive, the main features your doctor will look for which might indicate whether you are likely to miscarry subsequently are:

(i)    If your baby is growing normally but the amount of fluid around it in the pregnancy sac is very much reduced then there is a much higher chance of later miscarriage. If the pregnancy continues the volume will slowly increase over the next few weeks with no harm occurring to the baby.

(ii)   On the scan it is occasionally also possible to see some blood clot which would indicate where the bleeding has come from. If the amount of blood is small then it has no influence on the developing baby. If there is a large amount of blood clot present, however, there is an increased chance that you will miscarry subsequently. If clot is visible in your uterus you might later lose a small amount of old brown blood from your vagina. Most of it will absorb from within the uterus, however, just as a bruise absorbs elsewhere in the body.

(iii)  Rarely, the baby's heartbeat or its growth rate is too slow.

Occasionally other features about the pregnancy might be noted on the scan, such as where the placenta is developing, but in early pregnancy these do not appear to be of much consequence.

# ▌ CAUSES OF MISCARRIAGE

While this is really outside the scope of this book, your obstetrician will tell you that we rarely discover why your baby died. It is known that many or even most babies that die in early pregnancy do so because they had an abnormality, particularly of the chromosomes. The chance of it happening again in general is low. Many people wish to know the sex of the baby they have lost but as the death usually occurs very early in the pregnancy, this cannot be seen on ultrasound. For your own peace of mind you should recognize that it did not die because of anything you did; you could not have prevented it happening.

# ▌ PAIN IN EARLY PREGNANCY

Pain in pregnancy can be persistent and worrying to you. It is important to realize that pain is rarely the first sign of a miscarriage.

The first sign is bleeding and if pain occurs it is later, when the bleeding becomes heavy and the uterus contracts.

Pain in pregnancy unassociated with bleeding is very common but usually has no serious underlying cause. However, there are three important conditions that can cause pelvic pain early on which must be considered. Even when you have had no symptoms, these conditions may occasionally be suspected when your doctor feels a lump other than the pregnant uterus in the pelvis.

(i)     An **ectopic pregnancy** is one which develops outside the uterine cavity, the commonest type being inside the fallopian tube (figure 2.3). This can be a serious, even life-threatening, ordeal, as an ectopic pregnancy tends to rupture and bleed internally. While occasionally there are reports of a pregnancy in the abdomen resulting in a healthy baby, this is extraordinarily rare. Because of the dangers, surgery is undertaken as soon as the diagnosis is suspected.

An ectopic pregnancy may be suspected by your doctor if you develop pain in early pregnancy or because you are at special risk — perhaps you have had a previous ectopic pregnancy, pelvic infection, an operation on the fallopian tubes or infertility. This used to be a most difficult diagnosis for your doctor to make but with ultrasound it is much easier.

There are two ways of making this diagnosis with ultrasound. If the ultrasound is performed using a vaginal scanner, the ectopic pregnancy can usually be seen outside the uterus. If the scan is done through the abdomen, such a pregnancy will not usually be visible. In this case, the diagnosis is made when a woman known to be pregnant has no visible pregnancy inside the uterus. Such women will often need to have surgery to confirm the diagnosis, usually a laparoscopy — an examination of the inside of the abdomen with a medical telescope.

It is important to realize that ultrasound cannot *exclude* the possibility of an ectopic pregnancy. If a healthy pregnancy is inside the uterus you could also have an ectopic pregnancy, although this is extraordinarily rare. Alternatively, no matter how good the scanning equipment and the operator, a small ectopic pregnancy could be present but not picked up on the scan. With modern equipment, however, this is happening less often.

(ii)   Almost every woman in early pregnancy has an **ovarian cyst** known as the corpus luteum which forms in the ovary after the release of the egg. Thin-walled, the cyst is full of clear watery fluid and produces the hormones responsible for maintaining the pregnancy. It is generally small, between one and three centimetres in diameter, although occasionally it reaches five centimetres or more. The fluid in the cyst is usually absorbed over the first few months of pregnancy until it disappears totally. If there is a large cyst which persists after the first three months, an operation may occasionally be needed to remove it.

Occasionally ovarian cysts arise from other causes. On ultrasound, it is often possible to differentiate these from a corpus luteum. They may be larger, usually five centimetres in diameter or more, and often contain septa (or partitions) inside the fluid. They may also contain solid tissue instead of fluid. Most of these are not cancerous — it is very rare indeed to have an ovarian cancer in pregnancy. Despite this, it would usually be recommended that cysts containing solid areas be removed at around 14 weeks, or earlier if they are associated with severe pain.

(iii)   **Fibroids**, or fibromyomata to use their proper name, are thickenings of muscle and fibrous tissue in the wall of the uterus. These are very common, particularly in women over 40 years old (figure 2.3). They can reach a very large size, but they virtually never become cancerous. It is also very rare for them to interfere with the development or health of your baby. The main problems they present are first, that they may be difficult to diagnose and can be confused with an ovarian cyst, although usually they can be differentiated on ultrasound; second they may be a source of pain for you in the pregnancy. This may be of the greatest nuisance to you but still does not interfere with the baby's development. They are virtually never removed in pregnancy because the muscle of the uterus has such a rich blood supply that it would be difficult to control the bleeding. Very occasionally a fibroid low in the uterus may obstruct the birth of the baby.

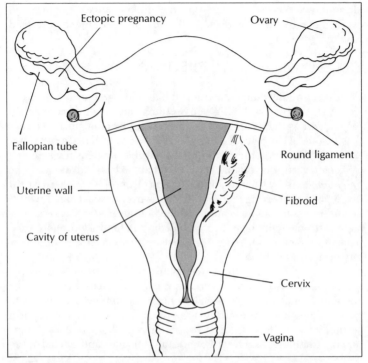

Fig 2.3 This diagram illustrates a non-pregnant uterus with the ovaries, fallopian tubes and round ligaments on each side. A fibroid is shown in the wall of the uterus. An ectopic pregnancy is illustrated in one tube.

# ▌ OTHER CAUSES OF PAIN

If you have pain and ultrasound shows a healthy pregnancy and no cyst or fibroid, then what is the cause? It may be due to a problem in your bowels or elsewhere but these are rarely detectable with ultrasound. If no cause is found then it is usually considered to be 'round ligament pain', due to stretching of the round ligament which helps support the uterus (see figure 2.3). If this is the cause of your pain then no abnormality is seen on ultrasound. The pain can be a nuisance over a moderately long period of the pregnancy, but it does ultimately settle down, usually in the middle stages. It causes no disturbance to the growth or well-being of the baby so you need have no fears.

# ▍BLEEDING IN LATE PREGNANCY

The causes of bleeding in the second half of pregnancy are different from those in the first half. When bleeding occurs in the second half, the concern is the location of the placenta. Bleeding after 20 weeks may be due to the placenta being too low in your uterus, a condition known as placenta praevia (figure 2.4). If this happens the bleeding is likely to recur, so you may have to remain in hospital and have the baby delivered by Caesarean section. Ultrasound is very accurate at diagnosing a low-lying placenta. It is, however, less accurate in diagnosing the other major cause of bleeding after 20 weeks, namely accidental haemorrhage. This is bleeding behind a normally sited placenta which if not severe or persistent should not require prolonged hospitalization.

Early in pregnancy the placenta often looks to be low in the uterus on ultrasound but becomes normally situated towards the end. How much notice is taken of it depends on how low it looks. In general, only if it is so low down that your doctor feels it will almost certainly remain low at the end of pregnancy, should it curtail some of your activities, such as long-distance travel and sexual intercourse.

# ▍Other Things Ultrasound can tell you

# ▍SEX OF THE BABY

'Can you tell what my baby is?' is the second most popular question pregnant women ask their sonographer. At first you may think this question is the same as 'Please tell me the sex of my baby'. It is not. Most pregnant women wish to know if the doctor can tell the sex but only some actually wish to know themselves. The decision as to when to find out the sex of the baby is of critical importance to families. Commonly one parent may wish to know and the other not. The one who decides against knowing may or may not be

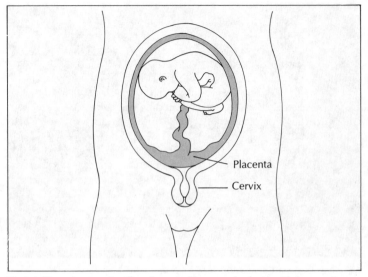

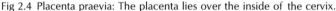

Fig 2.4 Placenta praevia: The placenta lies over the inside of the cervix.

happy for his or her partner to know. Many pregnant women appear most determined to find out the sex of their baby, but when told that the baby's sex cannot be seen are relieved. In addition, some obstetricians are happy for all their patients to find out the sex of their babies whilst others feel that this is not a good idea. In the middle of all these strong emotions sits the doctor performing the scan wondering what to do. If you and your partner do wish to know the sex, make this clear at the start of the scan.

There is no truth in the widely-held belief that the baby's heart rate tells you the sex. To determine the sex of a baby, the doctor looks at the genitals as shown in figures 2.5 and 2.6. The middle stage of pregnancy is the best time; by 20 weeks the sex of most babies can be seen but prior to 13 weeks it can be difficult. Towards the end of pregnancy, when there is less amniotic fluid around the baby in relation to the baby's size, it may again be hard to tell the sex. If the baby's back is uppermost (i.e. the baby is facing your spine), it is usually impossible to be sure.

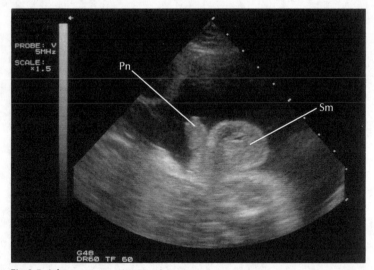

Fig 2.5 A boy: scrotum (Sm) and penis (Pn).

Fig 2.6 A girl: between the two thighs (Th) are the two female prominences, the labia (La) with the vagina visible between.

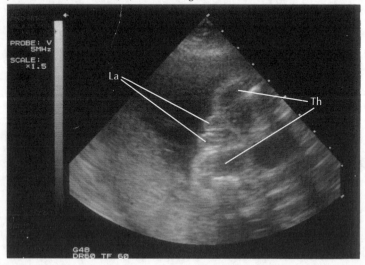

Do not count on the sex of the baby when seen on ultrasound as an absolute guarantee. It should, however, have an accuracy rate in the order of 98 per cent, depending on the stage of pregnancy, experience of the doctor and the position of the baby. Ask how confident the doctor is about the sex of your baby.

Occasionally couples ask to have the sex of their baby determined early on so they can have a termination if it is not what they want. Most doctors feel that this is an inappropriate use of a powerful technology also, by the time the doctor can be certain of the sex, the baby is likely to be too advanced for an abortion to be readily performed. In any case, most doctors would have difficulty accepting the sex of the baby as a legitimate ground for abortion, as it is a precedent for 'positive eugenics'.

# ■ GROWTH OF THE BABY

One of the main aims of obstetric care is to monitor your baby's growth. Your obstetrician would very much like to be able to calculate exactly your baby's weight before birth. How well your baby grows depends on the adequacy of the nutrition it receives across the placenta. If this is inadequate then it is at increased risk of a number of complications, including being stillborn. Growth assessment is usually done by your obstetrician palpating your abdomen, but if there are doubts about the growth an ultrasound examination may be ordered.

The aim of an ultrasound in this instance is to 'weigh' the baby. Clearly this is not possible before birth. Instead, two or three measurements are taken, particularly those of the baby's abdomen, head and femur. The likely birth weight is calculated from these measurements using charts. It cannot be precise, as the body build of babies, such as the amount of fat around their arms and legs, varies. It is, however, the best method available and will give a weight estimate to within 10 per cent accuracy approximately 75 per cent of the time. It will not of course tell you what its weight will be at birth — who can tell when your baby will deliver and what the growth will be like in the intervening period?

Using ultrasound there are features other than the baby's growth which may be assessed to determine its nutritional status. These include the amount of both the amniotic fluid present and fatty tissue it is laying down. As discussed in Chapter 1, looking at the placenta for signs of 'ageing' is not very helpful.

The purpose of monitoring the growth of your baby is to determine the optimal timing of delivery — to balance the risks of delivering it prematurely against those of leaving it undelivered. Only if your baby's growth is severely reduced would your obstetrician start to wonder if there could be an underlying genetic problem. Other tests may then be considered such as sampling the baby's blood for a chromosomal abnormality (which will be discussed in Chapter 10).

# ▍WELL-BEING OF THE BABY

One of the greatest challenges in obstetrics is to find a test which will show if the baby's well-being is suddenly jeopardized. Its growth may be measured on ultrasound every two weeks to check on nutrition, but what if its condition deteriorated rapidly? There are a number of tests available, none of which provide the whole answer. The most common use different sorts of ultrasound equipment, so we will look at them briefly.

(i)   **Cardiotocography** (CTG) is the most widely used test, providing a tracing of the baby's heartbeat for some 20 to 40 minutes. Specific clearly-defined variations in the heartbeat may indicate that the baby is in jeopardy.

(ii)  A **biophysical profile** provides a score to assess the baby's well-being. The movements of the baby's limbs, the 'breathing' movements and the amount of amniotic fluid around the baby are examined with ultrasound, and a CTG may also be performed. Not widely used in Australia, this is popular in North America and some other places. Babies who are in sudden distress tend to show no movements and there is usually a reduction in the amount of amniotic fluid around them.

(iii) **Fetal Doppler studies** involve the use of specially developed ultrasound equipment to check the patterns of your baby's blood flow through its blood vessels and umbilical cord (figure 2.7). These patterns change if placental function is reduced. This is a most interesting and exciting development but studies are still being carried out to test its efficacy in improving the outlook for babies.

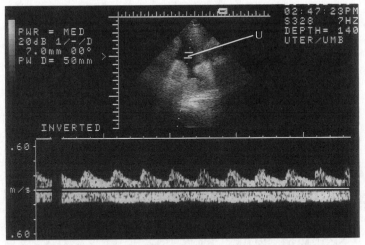

Fig 2.7 A Doppler examination of an artery of the umbilical cord (U) floating in amniotic fluid in the top half of the picture. The pulsations in the artery in the cord are visible in the lower half.

# ▌VARIATIONS IN THE AMOUNT OF AMNIOTIC FLUID

The amount of amniotic fluid around the baby may vary widely in normal situations. The reason for a little more or less than average is usually not known and is of no consequence. Occasionally, however, the amount of fluid is either much greater than or less than what is accepted as normal.

If there is an excess of fluid around the baby often no cause can be found, but it is likely to cause the mother increased discomfort. Occasionally it may be associated with a multiple pregnancy or an abnormality in the baby. Amniotic fluid is largely removed by the baby swallowing, so anything that prevents this, such as a blockage in the upper part of its intestine, can cause a fluid increase. Other causes include spina bifida, or a deficiency in the abdominal wall of the baby through which its intestines protrude (called exompholos). Most of these abnormalities can be seen on ultrasound, so if the baby appears normal in a scan, the likelihood is that there is no abnormality causing the increase. If there is a very large amount of fluid, your obstetrician might consider further testing such as fetal blood sampling or placental biopsy to exclude a chromosomal abnormality.

A reduction in the amount of fluid around your baby may be due to poor placental function. Your obstetrician would take extra care to watch the baby's growth. Occasionally there is no or minimal fluid around a baby. This may result from the baby not passing urine into the amniotic fluid due to inadequate or blocked kidney function or because of a severe reduction in blood flow through the placenta. (It might also be because your waters have broken but in this case you would usually be aware of fluid draining from the vagina.) A severe reduction in the amount of amniotic fluid may also be an indication for further testing of the baby.

# ▌ ULTRASOUND DOES NOT GUARANTEE A NORMAL BABY

Ultrasound is no panacea for obstetricians. Like any other test undertaken on your baby, it does not guarantee it will be normal. We all know a child may look totally normal and yet have some severe problems, such as mental retardation. Ultrasound is just a method of looking at a baby, albeit a more sophisticated method than merely looking at the features of a child after birth with the naked eye. With ultrasound we can see not only the parts of the baby which are visible after birth, like arms, legs and face, but also many of the internal organs. It is an excellent method for examining the structure of many of these organs but usually not their function. It can show in beautiful detail the structure of your baby's brain but it will tell you nothing of how well that brain works. If a baby is mentally retarded due to hydrocephaly (water on the brain) this will be seen on ultrasound, but unfortunately most mentally retarded babies have normal brain structure.

Remember that ultrasound can only detect abnormalities which are present at the time of the scan. Occasionally, abnormalities develop late in pregnancy, although most are present from a very early stage. Ultrasound is also not a good way of looking at adult bones. It cannot therefore tell if your pelvic size will be adequate for delivery.

# ▌Questions

WHERE HAS THE BLEEDING COME FROM?   This is often asked in relation to bleeding in early pregnancy. If a scan shows a blood clot in the uterus, outside but adjacent to the pregnancy sac, then this is where the bleeding has arisen. In the absence of such a clot it is impossible to know the source of bleeding but it is presumed to be somewhere adjacent to the developing placenta.

WILL THE BLEEDING DAMAGE THE BABY?   No. Bleeding in early pregnancy appears to cause few if any long-term problems for your baby. If you do not miscarry, then it should continue to develop normally.

WHEN DID MY BABY DIE?   This is commonly asked when a baby has died in early pregnancy. The crown-rump length of the baby gives a good indication of how advanced it was when it died. Parents like to work out what they were doing at the time of death to see what could have caused it. This is a fruitless task as the cause is almost always unknown and parents often blame inappropriately some innocuous event or activity.

I KNOW WHEN I CONCEIVED, SO WHY DOES THE SCAN GIVE A DIFFERENT DATE?   The first source of confusion is that obstetricians, for convenience take the beginning of pregnancy from the first day of the last period. If a woman feels she knows when she conceived she takes this as the beginning of pregnancy. A conversation with your doctor can usually resolve this difference.

If you are certain of your dates and a scan done in the first half of pregnancy differs from this date by more than a week then the scan is nearly always correct.

ARE THE DATES STILL CORRECT?   Couples often ask this after a second or subsequent scan. The earlier in pregnancy a scan is done the more accurate it is at predicting a due date. It would be inappropriate to change the date as a result of a scan done later in the pregnancy. A second scan is good at telling how the baby is growing but less precise at predicting a due date.

## WHEN WILL MY BABY BE BORN?
Ultrasound can give a very accurate due date, but of course nobody can tell if the baby will be born on that day. Some babies come very early and some very late. This unpredictable timing of the onset of labour is one of the mysteries of pregnancy.

## ARE MY TWINS JOINED?
In a multiple pregnancy each baby nearly always has its own separate bag of waters. If the membrane between the babies can be seen, and it nearly always can, this means that the babies could not be joined.

## ARE THE TWINS IDENTICAL?
The best way of working this out is by looking at the placenta and the membrane between the babies. If there are two placentas or the membrane is thick they are probably not identical. A single placenta occurs with identical twins but with non-identical twins the placentas may also be joined.

## WHAT DOES A LOW-LYING PLACENTA MEAN?
Early in pregnancy the placenta totally surrounds the pregnancy sac. By the end of the pregnancy the placenta occupies only a very small portion of the wall of the uterus. The placenta in early pregnancy therefore often looks low, but becomes normally sited later on. It takes experience to know how low a normal placenta can be at any particular stage of pregnancy. If there is any doubt, a second scan may be performed late in pregnancy to eliminate the possibility of placenta praevia.

## WILL WE KNOW THE SEX OF THE BABY?
It takes a great deal of experience to tell the sex of the baby and unless it is specifically pointed out you will not be able to see it. If you wish to know the sex, it is a good idea to mention this in advance. The genitals of the baby need to be closely examined to be sure of the sex, and usually the doctor will not do this unless specifically requested. It is sometimes possible to see the sex as early as 13 weeks and usually possible by 16 to 20 weeks.

## CAN YOU SEE HOW FAST THE BABY'S HEART IS BEATING?
Yes, you can always count the heartbeat. It is, however, very rarely of any consequence. Except in extreme circumstances, it

does not indicate how healthy the baby is. It does not even tell you what the sex is, despite many an old wives' tale.

## IS THE SIZE OF MY PELVIS NORMAL?    Ultrasound provides poor pictures of adult bones and is unable to tell you this.

## IS THE POSITION OF THE BABY CAUSING MY PAIN

In the first half of pregnancy lower abdominal pains are common. Pregnant women often blame the way the baby is lying, but this is an unlikely cause. Such pains may be due to a fibroid (a thickening of muscle and fibrous tissue in the wall of the uterus) or a cyst on the ovary. If neither of these are seen on ultrasound, the pain is often said to be caused by ligaments stretching. It produces no ill effects on the baby and will usually settle in mid-pregnancy.

## MY ULTRASOUND SUGGESTS THE PREGNANCY IS LESS ADVANCED THAN I EXPECTED; COULD IT BE THAT THE BABY IS NOT GROWING NORMALLY    It is

very rare for there to be significant alterations in growth of a baby in the first half of pregnancy. If there is poor growth, other signs, such as a reduced amount of amniotic fluid, are usually obvious. Hence, if your baby is significantly larger or smaller than expected prior to 20 weeks it is nearly always because you did not conceive at exactly the time you calculated.

## HOW LONG IS MY BABY?    As babies are curled up in the

uterus, the 'stretched out' length cannot be measured. Ultrasound will be used mostly to detect diameters, or bone lengths. The length of babies throughout pregnancy are shown in Chapter 1.

## IS MY BABY LYING THE CORRECT WAY?    Until the last

three months of pregnancy the baby's position varies. While the position of your baby is readily seen using ultrasound, a few minutes later it may change and this is quite normal. Most babies will remain head first from 34 weeks or earlier.

## WHY DOES THE BABY'S HEAD LOOK BIGGER THAN THE BODY?    The diameter of the head exceeds that of the body

throughout pregnancy until around 32 weeks. After 32 weeks fat starts to be deposited around the abdomen, which then becomes larger than the head.

# 3 THE ULTRASOUND EXAMINATION

This chapter will look at how ultrasound works and provide a step-by-step account of the examination. There is a great variety of ultrasound equipment in use. Many units are adequate for simple examinations, but not sufficiently sophisticated to allow diagnosis of most abnormalities. This chapter aims to show you different types of equipment and what they can do.

## What is Ultrasound?

A possible source of confusion is the many names used for the same test. As well as being called an ultrasound examination it is often referred to as a 'sonar' or 'scan' and may also be called an 'ultrasound scan', 'real-time scan', or 'sonar scan'. 'Scan' is really a loose term for any test which provides pictures of the inside of your body. In fact, methods other than ultrasound are rarely used for looking at a baby during pregnancy. Other imaging techniques provide less information about the baby, so any scan in pregnancy nearly always is ultrasound.

Ultrasound examinations use sound waves similar to those in our speech. Dog whistles use a frequency above the range of human hearing; ultrasound is a far higher frequency still. Humans can hear frequencies between about one and twenty thousand cycles per second, while ultrasound is usually one to twenty million cycles per second.

Sound waves we can hear travel readily in all directions through air. Ultrasound, however, has different properties. It does not travel

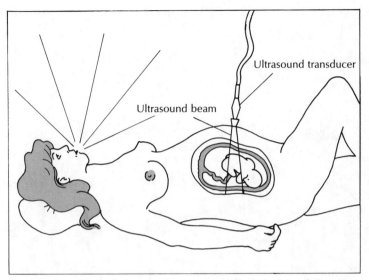

Fig 3.1 When we speak the sound waves travel through air in all directions whereas ultrasound uses sound waves, which travel through tissue but not air, and focus into a narrow beam like a beam of light.

through air, hence unless the transmitter actually touches you, no ultrasound reaches you. People watching the scan are therefore not exposed to any ultrasound.

Ultrasound also tends to travel in a straight line, and as shown in figure 3.1 can be made into a narrow beam like a torch light. Both the sound waves we hear and ultrasound have one important property in common — echoes occur when they hit an obstacle. Audible sound waves echo off a nearby wall or mountain, as shown in figure 3.2. Similarly, as ultrasound passes through the body echoes bounce off each tissue layer. It is these echoes which are registered by the machine to produce a picture.

# ▌How Ultrasound began

Ultrasound has been around longer than most people imagine, its medical use following development of the technology for other

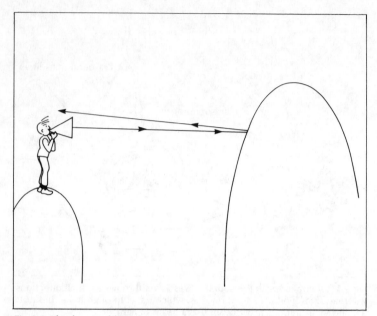

Fig 3.2 This boy is able to hear his voice echo from a distant mountain. In a similar way, ultrasound pictures are produced by transmitting sound waves through tissue which then echo back and are received, processed and displayed on a television screen.

purposes. The Allies first developed sonar during World War I for the detection of submarines. Industrial applications, such as flaw detection in metals followed. In 1948, the first primitive pictures of a baby prior to birth were produced, heralding ultrasound's entry into medicine. By the end of the 1950s it had been used for diagnosis of conditions in many parts of the body.

It was in obstetrics and gynaecology that ultrasound made the greatest early impact. Professor Ian Donald from Glasgow is acknowledged as the person who introduced ultrasound into clinical obstetrics in 1958. The first commercial ultrasound machine was available in 1963 and its use became widespread by the early 1970s. The beautifully detailed pictures we see today are a result of technological refinements made in the 1980s.

# Its use in Medicine

Ultrasound may be used to treat conditions as well as to diagnose them. It is widely used at much higher power levels than in obstetrics to speed the healing of injuries and even to break up kidney stones. It is also commonly used to diagnose conditions throughout the body in people of all ages. In this book we will concentrate on its use for producing pictures of babies.

Different types of ultrasound equipment are used in pregnancy. You may be surprised to learn that the 'microphone' used by obstetricians to listen to your baby's heartbeat when it cannot be heard by the stethoscope also uses ultrasound. Similarly, ultrasound equipment can trace your baby's heartbeat or be used to look at its blood flow when you are near the end of pregnancy.

# How the Ultrasound Machine works

This section can be skipped by those people who are not interested in how the ultrasound equipment operates.

If we were to run an electric current across a crystal (transducer) of a material like quartz or a ceramic substance, the energy would be converted into sound waves. These can be 'beamed' in a specific direction. As they traverse the body, they encounter various tissue interfaces from which they will be deflected back to the same transducer. This transducer then becomes a receiver and the sound waves are converted back into electric pulses. The machine takes the electrical information provided by the echoes and transforms it into a two-dimensional picture on a television monitor.

The pulses of sound are short, approximately one millionth of a second. They are fired about a thousand times per second. We can therefore already see one of the safety factors in the equipment — if the ultrasound machine is applied for one second, sound waves are only being applied for one thousandth of a second. The rest of the time is spent receiving the echoes between pulses. So if your examination takes thirty minutes (1800 seconds), then the ultrasound is only actively working for 1.8 seconds.

One of the great advances in the 1980s was the development of 'real-time' ultrasound equipment. 'Real-time' means that moving pictures are produced of your baby instead of the old still ones. There are many ways that these moving pictures can be produced, and the methods are not important here, but they have one thing in common — they produce images of sections, or slices, of tissue (figure 3.3).

If the section is taken up and down a pregnant woman's abdomen then the inside of her abdomen in the long axis of her body is shown on the screen. In the figure shown, the baby is lying head down along the long axis of the mother so the slice shows the whole length of the baby. As it is a slice, all of the baby is never on the same picture — if the head and body are on the screen, the limbs will usually not be visible. In addition, since it is a slice, the insides of the baby are visible, allowing its heart and other internal organs to be seen on the screen. It is like slicing a loaf of bread and examining each slice in turn. The doctor can magnify part of the baby so that none of the mother's tissues are visible on the screen.

As well as enabling us to *see* tissues, ultrasound makes it possible to take very accurate *measurements*. It is known that ultrasound travels through tissues at approximately 1540 metres per second. The machine measures how long it takes for sound waves to travel to a point, such as the baby's leg, and back. It can be designed to read out how far that leg is from the transducer since

distance = time (which the machine knows) × speed of ultrasound (1540 metres per second)

Modern ultrasound machines use electronic calipers which the operator freely moves around the television monitor to allow the distance between any two points to be accurately measured.

Despite the sophistication of modern ultrasound equipment, there are two features people often enquire about which are not available. The first is colour pictures. For colour to be of value it must provide additional information which helps diagnosis. It would also be preferable if the colours were lifelike. This has only been successful in certain specialized areas such as the examination of blood flowing in vessels and is not widely used in pregnancy. The second enquiry is whether engineers will develop three-dimensional ultrasound instead of the two-dimensional sections. Vast amounts of work have gone into development and although success has been

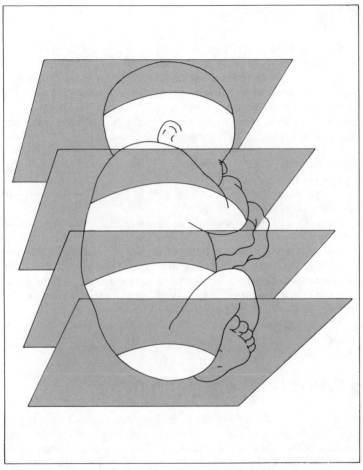

Fig 3.3 An ultrasound picture cannot show all of the baby at once, but shows one section (or slice) through one part of the baby at a time, similar to one of the sections shown here.

achieved, it is unlikely to be in widespread use in the near future. Our pictures, for some time, are likely to remain black and white (and grey) and in two dimensions.

# The Equipment

Anybody who had an ultrasound examination more than five years ago and then another one since could not help but notice that the equipment has been reduced in size. Early equipment used to fill half a moderate-sized room while the modern version (figure 3.4) is a relatively small unit sitting beside the couch. At the same time, there has been an increase in the range of transducers and a great improvement in the quality (or resolution) of the images. Ultrasound machines are now large computers with sophisticated software. Meanwhile, the price has unfortunately also increased, with some equipment now costing several times as much as the average house. Such equipment may only be available in regional centres and at specialist practices.

Small, cheaper equipment is widely available and is useful for basic work such as detecting twins and measuring the head size to calculate dates. To make the large number of more difficult diagnoses that are possible with ultrasound requires sophisticated (and expensive) state-of-the-art equipment. You may find it difficult to recognize such equipment; one way of assessing the level of sophistication of the kind used by your doctor would be to ask if it was good for diagnosing such structural abnormalities as spina bifida.

# Who should perform the Scan?

As important as the quality of the equipment is the expertise of the operator. When you have your ultrasound examination you will want to know that it is being performed by an expert. As a rule of thumb, if the aim of the scan is to thoroughly check the baby for abnormalities, more than 750 examinations a year should be made to maintain experience. The scan may be carried out by your own doctor, by a specialist or by a technician known as a sonographer. In the latter case, the pictures are later interpreted and reported by the doctor. All methods can work well with appropriately trained and experienced personnel. Many ultrasound courses and examinations are available. For some of the more simple examinations, such as

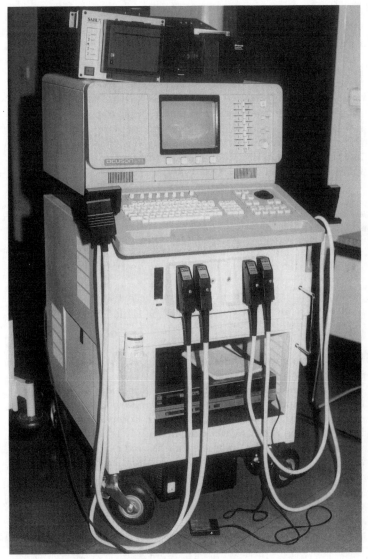

Fig 3.4  A modern ultrasound machine.

checking the heartbeat or the position of the baby, less examinations are needed. Experience in looking at babies prior to birth is at least as important as the qualifications a person holds.

# Can Ultrasound damage your Baby?

There have been hundreds of scientific reports published on the safety of ultrasound and none have found any reproducible ill effects. The Australian Society for Ultrasound in Medicine, whose brief is to continuously watch the scientific literature, published the following statement in August 1988 :

> Diagnostic ultrasound has been in clinical use since the late 1950s. To date the results of numerous follow-up studies on patients and children who have been examined before birth have failed to demonstrate any biological effect which could be attributed to the ultrasound examination.
>
> Given the known benefits and demonstrated efficacy of the medical diagnosis, the Australian Society for Ultrasound in Medicine considers that the prudent use of diagnostic ultrasound far outweighs the risks, if any, that may be present. There is no reason to withhold the application of the technique when it is indicated on clinical grounds.

Similar statements have been produced by equivalent organizations in other countries.

Research into the effects of ultrasound includes laboratory studies of cell changes, animal research, and follow-up studies of babies exposed to ultrasound. In each case no reproducible ill effects have been shown to result. A well-designed study reported in 1984 involved 425 babies who underwent ultrasound examination prior to birth and 381 matched controls, babies of similar background who were not scanned. Physical development and tests of nerve function were compared at birth and again between seven and twelve years, revealing no significant differences.

One of the most widely publicized adverse reports was of changes in the chromosomes of cells exposed to ultrasound. This report has not been confirmed by other workers using the same methods, so it is believed that the reported chromosome changes must have been caused by some other agent. While there has been criticism of the construction of some studies, the sheer number showing no ill effect has reassured physicists, obstetricians and radiologists that ultrasound examinations are safe. Confidence in its safety has reached such a level that it has become a routine procedure in pregnancy in many countries. Indeed, in Germany the law demands that every pregnant woman must be offered two ultrasound examinations by her doctor — one early in pregnancy and one late.

There are several factors which reduce the possibility of harm from ultrasound. When examining a pregnancy, low power levels are used. In the previous section we explained that ultrasound uses extremely short pulses of sound, so that the transducer is only sending out sound waves for approximately one thousandth of the examination time. You will also see only part of your baby on the screen at one time, so the rest of it is receiving minimal ultrasound exposure. Thus any one part of the baby receives ultrasound for a very short time during the examination.

It has been known for a long time that ultrasound at much higher power levels than is used for diagnosis can produce cell damage. These high power levels have been used for the treatment of cancer and by physiotherapists to treat muscle injuries. They should not be directed at the abdomen of a pregnant woman.

Despite its safety record, ultrasound should not be used unnecessarily; it is recommended for clinical benefit only. Most people would feel that to have an ultrasound examination merely to find out the sex of the baby would be frivolous. If, however, a scan is being carried out for some other reason then it takes little extra time to look at the sex if that is the parents' wish.

Neither you nor your baby will notice any sensation from your ultrasound examination. In particular, the scan does not make you feel warm. As you do not feel anything, and you receive more power than your baby since the ultrasound must pass through your tissues first, your baby also cannot feel anything. Ultrasound cannot make your baby move. Any movements observed during the examination are those that would have occurred naturally. There has also never been any evidence to support the suggestion that ultrasound can damage your baby's hearing.

# ▌The Examination

The most vivid memories many women have of the scan is of an agonizingly full bladder. Fortunately this is now rarely necessary. An overfull bladder is in fact counterproductive, usually resulting in poor pictures. Check what your doctor wants you to drink. Often a little urine in your bladder is preferred but sometimes a totally empty one is best.

The logic of a full bladder was that it lifts the uterus out of your pelvis, sometimes making it easier to see through the abdomen. It also pushes the bowel away from in front of the uterus. As bowel contains air through which ultrasound will not pass, its presence results in poor images. Modern equipment allows the doctor to obtain good views without a full bladder by angling a small transducer through a part of the abdomen where intestines are not in the way.

When you lie on the examination couch for your ultrasound examination, some gel is squirted onto your abdomen — if you are lucky it will be warm. This gel allows the ultrasound to travel into your abdomen from the transducer. Without the gel there would be a thin layer of air between your skin and the transducer which would reflect the ultrasound. As the transducer rests or is only pressed gently on your abdomen, it will not hurt. It is moved around to produce images of sections through different parts of the baby. At the completion of the scan the gel is wiped off.

If you need a scan in late pregnancy, you may have difficulty lying for a long period on your back. You may develop backache, simply feel uncomfortable or may become faint, dizzy, hot and sweaty. This is because the baby and its amniotic fluid press on the blood vessels returning blood to your heart from your legs. If this happens then tell the doctor — it is best to turn onto your side and you will quickly feel better.

## ▌VAGINAL SCAN

This type of scan is also known as transvaginal (which means through the vagina) or endovaginal (which means in the vagina). A special transducer is gently passed into the vagina as you lie on your back with your legs bent up (see figure 3.5). The transducer, with its

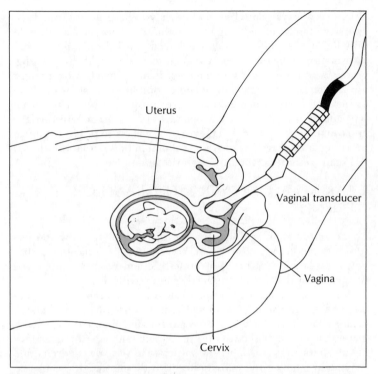

Fig 3.5 A vaginal scan: the transducer is passed into the vagina and 'looks through' the walls of the vagina and uterus at the baby. Note that the transducer does not pass into the cervix or uterus, so it cannot disturb the pregnancy.

disposable cover, sits in the vagina, not in the uterus so it can in no way harm a pregnancy or increase the risk of miscarriage. The transducer is cleaned after each use and wrapped in a clean disposable cover for each patient so there is no risk of developing AIDS or other infections from the examination. A vaginal scan does not hurt — most transducers are similar in size to one finger so cause less discomfort than a gynaecological examination. Some people would prefer to pass the scanner themselves and there is no reason why you should not do this if you wish.

At first the idea of this scan is unpleasant and sounds uncomfortable. It is always your choice whether you have it performed. Of course you may refuse a vaginal scan but don't forget that it would only be suggested if the doctor believed that it would allow more information to be obtained. A vaginal scan is more likely to be suggested if you are in early pregnancy. It has proved to be a major advance in the management of some complications allowing them to be diagnosed earlier than was previously possible. It has been particularly useful in the early diagnosis of threatened miscarriage and tubal (or ectopic) pregnancy. You are likely to be given a much more accurate diagnosis of your problem in these situations than if the scan were performed through the abdomen.

# ▋ TAKING ALONG YOUR HUSBAND OR FRIEND

Check before your scan that the doctor is happy to show you features of your baby on the screen. You should also indicate whether you are planning to bring in your husband or other interested people. Most doctors are perfectly happy with this.

While many parents wish to include other children in the experience of the first look of your baby, this is not always successful. Children under twelve years of age cannot understand the scan with its two-dimensional 'slice of information' and may become restless. Finally, a warning — you will be surprised how many children think they will be taking the baby home with them after the scan.

# ▋ INTERPRETATION OF THE PICTURE

You will find the scan an exciting and rewarding experience but don't expect to understand every picture. Some views, such as a profile shot of your baby, are very straightforward, but others will be difficult or impossible for the inexperienced eye to interpret. You must keep in mind that you are looking at sections of your baby and so will see the internal organs, not just the external appearance. A cross-section of the head is therefore not a view from above but rather a circle — the skull — with the inside of the brain visible within.

It takes years of practice to be able to fully interpret ultrasound pictures. You will mostly understand only the features pointed out to you. It is impossible for the doctor to point out everything as well as concentrate on assessing the baby's development. While doctors are aware that one of the joys of the ultrasound examination is that it enables you to relate to your unborn baby, it is also important as the first medical check.

The picture is nearly always presented as white on a black background. Solid tissue, such as bones, is seen as densely white, soft tissue as a lighter grey, and water or fluid as black. Hence the skull and long bones of the arms and legs are easy to see. The baby's bladder (which contains urine), the stomach (which contains fluid swallowed from the amniotic cavity) and blood in the heart look black. The amniotic fluid around the baby also looks black (see figures 4.2–4.8).

As you look at the screen, the top of the picture is your skin and the bottom is deep into your body. The left of the picture may be your left or right, head or feet end, depending on which way the transducer is orientated. The picture can be magnified, with centimetre marks down the side of the screen indicating the size of the picture in relation to actual size. In general what you see on the screen is beneath where the transducer touches you — if you see the head when the transducer is low on your abdomen then the head is lowermost in your body (figure 3.6).

If your baby is facing upwards, the doctor can show you a lifelike profile view (figure 3.7). If, however, it is facing away towards your spine, the face is hard to see and the picture looks much less like a real human being.

Strangely you will find you can see much more human-looking pictures of your baby earlier in pregnancy. At 10 or 12 weeks your tiny fetus usually will lie face up and the pictures can be quite beautiful. At 16 to 20 weeks wonderfully lifelike pictures of most babies can also usually be obtained. In the last three months of pregnancy, however, you are likely to be disappointed and find you cannot make out nearly as much detail (figure 3.8). At that time your baby is too large for its entire image to fit onto the screen at one time. Each picture represents a thin slice of information from only a part of your baby's anatomy and is thus hard for you to interpret.

Your own body build will alter the quality of the pictures. If you are plump the layer of fat between your baby and the transducer

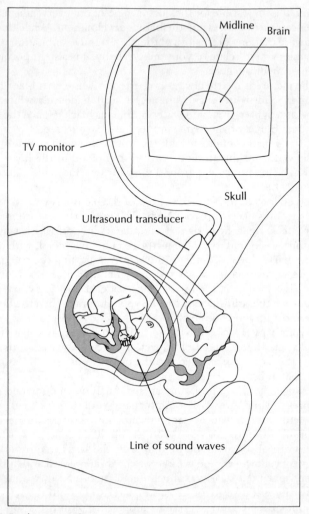

Fig 3.6 Producing an ultrasound picture: the ultrasound transducer sends out a line of sound waves through the tissues of the mother and baby. Small echoes from tissue layers reflect back to the transducer and are imaged on a TV monitor. As the transducer is over the baby's head a section (or slice) through the head is displayed — inside the skull, the brain and midline between the two halves of the brain are seen.

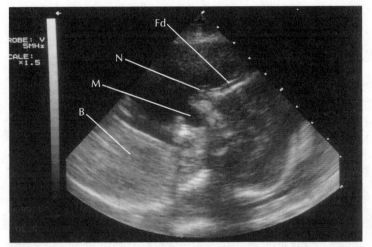

Fig 3.7 A profile view of a baby showing forehead (Fd) nose (N) mouth (M) and body (B).

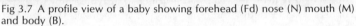

Fig 3.8 In the last three months of pregnancy the baby is too large to be seen on one picture. With some machines a composite picture such as shown here can be produced showing the head (H) with the line separating the two brain hemispheres, ribs (R) and body on the left.

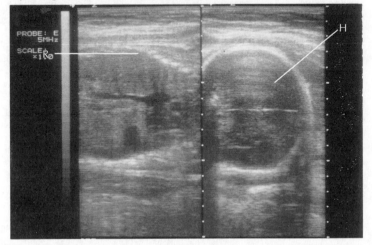

may prevent good pictures being obtained. Scars on your abdomen can also cause poor contact and result in poor pictures. Finally, the skill of the operator and the quality of the equipment will affect the clarity of the images.

# ❚ A PICTURE TO TAKE HOME

'May I have a picture?' is undoubtedly the most frequent question asked. The answer is nearly always 'yes'. In this section we will look at the type of pictures available for you to take home with you and also for the doctor's medical records (figure 3.9).

The first method introduced was polaroid film, and this still provides the most convenient, best-quality, longest-lasting picture of your baby. It remains widely used but unfortunately is expensive. Although the picture lasts well it does not last indefinitely and over ten years or so it does start to fade. These pictures may be readily copied by any professional photographer to provide you with extra copies for other family members and one for yourself that will last indefinitely.

To overcome the cost of polaroid film, thermal printers have been introduced. These pictures are very cheap. They are produced on glossy thin paper so look less like a 'real' picture. The image is also not as high a quality as on polaroid film. These are unsatisfactory for your long-term record of your unborn baby because they fade with time especially if exposed to light. Both the image quality and the life of these pictures are, however, improving.

The third option for a still record of your baby is a film similar to that used for X-rays. This is good for the doctors' records — high-quality, long-lasting, relatively cheap images — but not as acceptable to you for your baby's first photograph. When showing a clinical X-ray type picture of your baby to friends and relatives, it must be held up to the light.

Those looking for the ultimate record may desire a videotape of their unborn baby. The idea is often better than the reality — without somebody to point out the details to you later, this mass of cross-sectional images of your baby's insides may mean little to you and your friends at a later date. There is some resistance to video-tapes amongst doctors on several scores. It requires much more organization than a simple snapshot — a second video recorder (if

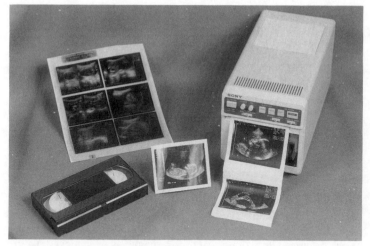

Fig 3.9 The types of pictures which can be produced using ultrasound —
Polaroid picture, X-ray film, video, thermal printer.

the doctor uses one for his own records) or a constant change of
tapes for successive patients. The provision of tapes may be difficult
if the patient forgets to bring one. Finally, it should be pointed out
that with so many distractions (taking a video tape for the family,
recording pictures for the medical record, showing the pregnant
woman and her family and friends on the screen), many doctors are
worried that mistakes are more likely in the most important area —
a check of the baby.

# ▌Questions

IS THAT RINGING SOUND THE ULTRASOUND
WAVES?    The noise that you hear is not the ultrasound waves.
Some transducers make a ringing noise but this is machine noise.
Ultrasound waves cannot be heard — they are above the range of
human hearing.

IS ULTRASOUND AN X-RAY?    No, there are no X-rays used

during an ultrasound examination. Ultrasound involves sound waves only. These are similar to those of speech so they do not have the potential problems of X-rays.

## DO THE SOUND WAVES MAKE THE BABY MOVE?
Even though you might only be seeing the baby on the screen, the sound waves have in fact passed through you first. You receive far more of the ultrasound power than the baby. Neither you nor the baby feel anything nor does the ultrasound stimulate movement. Those movements you see on the screen are the natural movements of the baby in the uterus. Usually during the course of any scan after 9 weeks you will see at least some movements of your baby.

## DOES ULTRASOUND HURT THE BABY'S EARS?    No ill effects of ultrasound have been found at the levels used for diagnosis. Doctors would not do the scan if it damaged the baby's ears or other organs. Ultrasound used for diagnosis is believed to be safe.

## MUST I HAVE A VAGINAL SCAN?    It is always your option to say no to any medical treatment which is offered to you. Usually a vaginal scan would only be offered if it is likely to provide better information. This is most likely to happen early in pregnancy.

## IS THAT CIRCLE A PICTURE OF THE BABY'S HEAD FROM ABOVE?    As shown in figure 4.2, the picture is not taken from above but represents thin slices of tissue. The circle therefore represents an image of the skull around the outside with the softer echoes of the brain within. It is as if you sliced through the baby's head and looked at the sliced end.

## WHY IS MY PICTURE NOT AS GOOD AS THAT OF MY FRIENDS?    The picture you are given depends on the stage of pregnancy and the way the baby is facing. A profile view can be obtained that produces the most human-looking image but this is not always possible. It also applies that the better the ultrasound machine, the better the picture is likely to be.

CAN YOU STILL SEE THROUGH THE BABY?   When they see inside their baby on ultrasound, some people have the misconception that fetuses in early pregnancy are transparent. While they do have thin skin, you cannot see through them. Just as ultrasound travels through your tissues to get to the baby, so it also travels through the baby's skin to provide an image of its insides.

WHERE ARE THE ARMS AND LEGS ON MY PICTURE?
A picture for you to keep is usually taken to include the baby's head and body. It is not possible to include all the arms and legs in the same slice.

CAN I LISTEN TO THE BABY'S HEARTBEAT?   Ultrasound equipment can be designed with a speaker so you can hear your baby's heartbeat. The equipment used to examine your pregnancy produces a picture on a television monitor so you can see the heartbeat but not hear it.

# 4 WHAT ULTRASOUND CAN SHOW YOU

The aim of this chapter is to indicate which structures in your baby may be visualized with ultrasound. We will concentrate on those structures which are felt to be important by pregnant women and are often asked about, as well as those that are important medically because of the frequency or significance of abnormalities in that area. As you are having your ultrasound examination, remember that each normal structure seen excludes or reduces the risk of an abnormality in that area. For example, if you are shown a section of the spine which has a normal appearance then a spina bifida is unlikely in that area.

## What Abnormalities are looked for?

Irrespective of the reasons for your ultrasound examination, it is normal to examine the entire pregnancy — the baby, amniotic fluid and placenta — as well as the uterus, and also your pelvis for lumps. Areas which are particularly relevant to your situation are always examined in special detail, such as the baby's spine if you have previously had a baby with spina bifida.

It should be emphasized that not all abnormalities can be detected with ultrasound. Ultrasound shows structures which can be quite normal but the organ may still be disordered in function: for example, mental retardation commonly occurs in infants who have a normally structured brain. The contrary also holds, in that the structure may appear grossly abnormal, but produce only minor difficulties to the baby after birth. For example, a baby with exomphalos (or a defect in its abdominal wall) may have a large structural abnormality but after birth a simple operation will result in a perfectly normal child. Some very mild defects may indicate a more severe abnormality elsewhere; for example, a baby with overriding fingers may have a chromosomal abnormality.

Which abnormalities can be detected at an ultrasound examination depend greatly on the stage at which the pregnancy is scanned, and any technical difficulties encountered at the time. Unfortunately, an abnormality which is readily diagnosed if the baby is lying in one position may be difficult or impossible to diagnose if it is facing the opposite direction. A small heart abnormality or a cleft lip may be visible if the baby faces up but not if it faces down. In the best hands, however, ultrasound can detect an abnormality in up to 1 per cent of babies. It can detect in fact a wider range than is detectable by the more invasive tests such as amniocentesis and CVS.

# When is the Best Time?

Eighteen weeks is often chosen as the best time for an ultrasound examination because:

(i)     it is early enough to enable the due date to be calculated with sufficient accuracy in most pregnancies;

(ii)    at this time the baby is far enough advanced for most normal structures to be clearly visible;

(iii)   if an abnormality is discovered it is early enough to have an abortion if this is the parents' wish.

Eighteen weeks is not the best time for an ultrasound examination for everybody. Women who have a complication either of this pregnancy or a previous one may well have an ultrasound examination much earlier. Those who have previously delivered a baby with hydrocephaly (water on the brain) or dwarfism may have an ultrasound examination a little later, as their measurements may remain within normal limits at 18 weeks.

# Why is a Scan so Important?

Obstetricians are increasingly recommending that an ultrasound examination to check the structure of the baby be carried out during pregnancy. The advantages of doing so are as follows:

(i)   It provides enormous reassurance to parents. Most parents worry a great deal about the normality of their baby during pregnancy. The reassurance of seeing normal structures, plus the added bonding that a normal ultrasound examination provides, is reason enough for the examination for many people.

(ii)  If a significant abnormality is present, a couple may decide to have the pregnancy terminated. Couples who decide to continue the pregnancy have the advantage of being forewarned of the abnormality.

(iii) The knowledge that an abnormality is present allows medical staff to be forewarned. Some of the abnormalities detected on ultrasound may require urgent treatment at birth if the baby is to have the best chance of healthy survival. This often means that delivery should take place at a hospital where specialists and paediatric facilities are available.

(iv)  It is sometimes important to know than an abnormality is present to allow a delivery to be brought on early, thus helping to minimize the continuing damage from that abnormality prior to birth. If ultrasound detects blocked kidneys, for example, and the condition deteriorates, the baby would be delivered early and the disease treated.

(v)   There are occasional, albeit rare, abnormalities which may be treated prior to birth. Some of these are described in Chapter 10.

# Minor Abnormalities

The sensitivity of ultrasound equipment now enables many minor variations from the norm to also be detected. Unfortunately it is difficult to convince a couple whose unborn child is shown to have an abnormality that it will only be minor. It is very difficult as a parent to keep such a finding in perspective. The widespread belief today that it is the parent's right to be fully informed of even the most minor abnormality can produce heightened parental anxiety over an insignificant defect. Some of the minor abnormalities which are relatively commonly identified on ultrasound, such as mis-shapen (club) feet and mild hydronephrosis (fluid on the kidneys) will be discussed in this section. For a more complete discussion on the structure and abnormalities which can occur in a developing baby, *Prenatal Diagnosis of Congenital Anomalies* by Romero, Filu, Jeanty, Ghidini and Hobbins is recommended.

# ▌Down Syndrome

As most babies with Down syndrome have no major structural abnormalities, the condition cannot readily be detected on ultra-sound. There are some subtle facial differences, but again these are not generally picked up with a scan. The baby may however, have heart abnormalities or a blockage in the upper part of the intestines which may sometimes be identified. In such cases, it may be sug-gested that the baby's chromosomes be tested to exclude the presence of Down syndrome.

Efforts have been made to discover more subtle signs of the syndrome. The first suggested was that the baby's head was more likely to be circular in shape, rather than the elongated shape of a normal skull. This has not proven to be a useful sign. A second sign which may be associated with Down syndrome is very slight extra thickening of the skin and soft tissue at the back of the skull. While some babies with Down syndrome do have this sign, others do not and it is uncertain how often it is present in the normal population. If a baby does have minor swelling at the back of its neck and is shown not to have Down syndrome, then it in no way affects its future development. A further subtle sign of Down syndrome sug-gested has been that the femur is slightly shorter than expected. The usefulness of this as a test for screening is uncertain. Finally a baby with Down syndrome may have minor abnormalities of the little finger. The bone centre in the middle section of the 5th finger may be smaller than expected, and the 5th finger may overlap the 4th finger. Again it is uncertain how often this sign will be detected on ultrasound. In all, some babies with Down syndrome may be picked up on ultrasound but the proportion remains unknown. There is no sign observable using ultrasound which will say for certain that a baby does have Down syndrome. These signs merely raise the index of suspicion — confirmation requires CVS, amniocentesis or fetal blood sampling to assess the chromosomes.

# ▌Ultrasound Sections

Ultrasound is used to make a series of sections through the baby to visualize various structures and organs. The diagram in figure 4.1 shows where each of the ultrasound sections is taken.

## ▌HEAD AND SPINE

Figure 4.2 shows a section high up in the head with the skull encasing the brain. Note that it is a slice through the tissues of the skull and brain so that the structure of the brain itself is visible. It is not a view from above the head. This section is carefully examined as it contains the midline between the two halves of the brain, as well as the lateral ventricles which are the main fluid-containing chambers. Three important abnormalities can be picked up in this section.

**Anencephaly** is a condition in which the bony skull and most of the brain is absent. It is readily identified as the structures normally seen in the section through the head and brain are all missing. There is of course no possible treatment and the baby dies before or immediately after birth. The incidence of anencephaly varies throughout the world between 1 and 2 per 1000. It is slightly higher in Ireland and Wales and lower in Asian countries.

**Hydrocephaly** is an increase in the amount of cerebrospinal fluid in the chambers of the brain. Occurring in 0.5 to 3 births per thousand, this is diagnosed when the size of the ventricles is larger than expected. Hydrocephaly is often associated with other abnormalities and is present at birth in nearly all babies with spina bifida. After birth hydrocephaly is treated by placing a tube (a shunt) from the enlarged ventricles to the abdomen to drain the fluid. Prior to birth, hydrocephaly can be treated by a drainage procedure but the results of this technique suggest that it does little to reduce the damage from the condition. The outlook for hydrocephaly depends

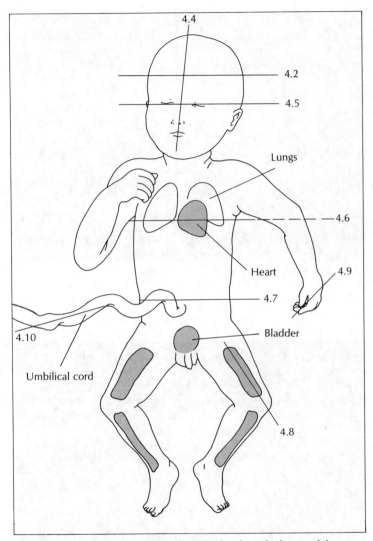

Fig 4.1 Each of the lines corresponds to the level at which one of the ultrasound images discussed and illustrated in this chapter was taken.

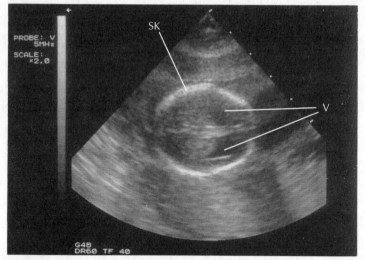

Fig 4.2 The head, showing the fluid-filled chambers of the brain
(V=ventricle) and the midline which separates the two hemispheres of the
brain (Sk=skull).

Fig. 4.3 The two parallel lines form the bones of the spine (Sp) with the
skin (Sn) overlying it.

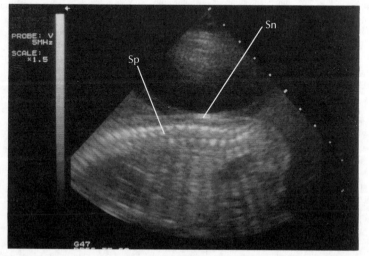

on its cause and severity. Severe hydrocephaly detected prior to birth has a very poor outlook.

**Choroid plexus cysts** lie adjacent to the ventricles in the tissue which produce the cerebro-spinal fluid. Occurring in about 1 per cent of babies prior to birth they are readily diagnosed when a small fluid collection of up to 2 cm in diameter is seen adjacent to the ventricle. Taken alone, these are not serious — most cysts disappear during the course of pregnancy — but it has been suggested that they are associated with an increased incidence of Trisomy 18. This is a severe chromosomal abnormality in which the baby usually dies prior to or shortly after birth. If a choroid plexus cyst is found, and especially if there are several large cysts, it is therefore important that a careful examination be performed to look for other abnormalities associated with Trisomy 18.

A section of the whole length of the spine can be seen in figure 4.3. It normally shows each of the vertebra bodies and the overlying skin. In the presence of **spina bifida**, there is usually a lack of skin and an absence of the back wall of the vertebrae in the affected segment of the spine. This condition is covered in greater detail in the following chapter.

# ▌ FACE AND NECK

In figure 4.4 the baby's nose, lips and chin are visible in profile. Figure 4.5 shows the baby's eyes and the bridge of its nose. A lower section will show the line of the upper jaw, the overlying lip, and at the back, the lower part of the skull in the region of the back of the neck.

The face of the baby is examined to assess the size of the eye sockets and the features of the baby's profile and mouth. **Facial clefts** are the most common abnormality in this area, estimated to occur in approximately 1 per 1000 births. Most of these involve the lip alone or the lip and the underlying palate. If the palate alone is affected it is usually at the back, so it is unlikely to be diagnosed on ultrasound. With satisfactory views of the baby's face, many of those with a large cleft lip and palate may be detected, but the smaller lesions may be difficult or impossible to see. They are diagnosed on ultrasound when a deficiency in the line of the upper lip is seen. If this is the only abnormality then a good cosmetic result can be expected with current surgical techniques.

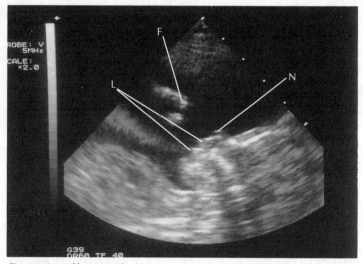

Fig 4.4 A profile view of a baby showing nose (N) lips (L) and fingers (F) in front of the face.

Fig 4.5 A section across the face showing the eyes (E) and bridge of the nose (N). A hand (Ha) is seen to the left.

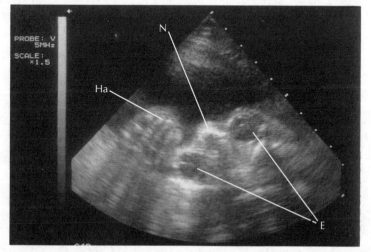

**Cystic swellings** around the neck of the baby occur in approximately 1 in 200 pregnancies that miscarry but are uncommon in liveborn babies. These are readily diagnosed on ultrasound by noting the swellings themselves. The outlook for the baby depends on the degree of swelling of the neck and elsewhere in the baby's body. This condition may indicate a chromosomal abnormality, most likely Turner syndrome (see Chapter 5).

## ▌ HEART AND LUNGS

In the cross-section of the baby's chest shown in figure 4.6 the four chambers of the heart are visible. If other sections are also taken around the heart then the vessels entering and leaving the heart may also be examined.

There are a large number of structural abnormalities of the heart and they occur in at least one in 125 births. Many of these are not detectable prior to birth. This is a difficult area of diagnosis that requires equipment with excellent resolution and an experienced

Fig 4.6 A section across the chest showing the four heart chambers and septum (Se) separating the right and left sides of the heart. The lungs are to either side of the heart. (Sp=spine, Cs=front of chest wall).

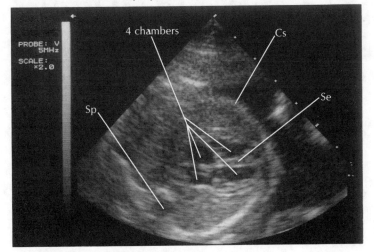

operator. Under these conditions, however, it is now possible to detect at 18 weeks almost half of those babies with a heart abnormality. Advances in cardiac surgery have meant that babies who would have previously died of the heart abnormality may now be treated surgically after birth. If a heart abnormality is detected with ultrasound it is usually recommended that the chromosomes of the baby be tested.

Abnormalities of the lungs prior to birth are rare. The most common is a cyst on one lung which is diagnosed when a localized fluid collection is seen beside the heart. Even if quite large, these may often be removed after birth with an excellent outlook for the baby. Occasionally they need to be drained prior to birth.

# ABDOMEN AND ABDOMINAL WALL

The section shown in figure 4.7 is the most important one for checking the growth of the baby. Deficiencies in the skin and muscle of the abdominal wall may lead to some of the contents developing outside the abdomen. There are two conditions: **exomphalos** where there is a lining over the bulge and **gastroschisis**, where there is none. Together these occur in approximately 1 in 5000 births. They are usually readily diagnosed on ultrasound and require no treatment prior to birth. Most can be closed after birth with a most successful outcome. Some of the babies with an exomphalos may also have other associated abnormalities which may be detected with ultrasound or by chromosomal analysis.

**Diaphragmatic hernia** is a deficiency in the baby's diaphragm so that some of the contents of the abdomen ride up into the chest. The hernia is most commonly on the left side of the diaphragm with the stomach becoming positioned in the chest. This type is often diagnosed on ultrasound but some of the other types are more difficult. The hernia can be surgically treated at birth, but the major problem in these babies is that the presence of abdominal contents in the chest constricts the growth of the lungs. This is difficult to test prior to birth, but after birth it may be found that the lung development is inadequate for the baby's survival.

**Kidney abnormalities**. The kidneys represent one of the more difficult diagnostic areas. While they may be seen early in pregnancy it is their function which is of prime importance. This is

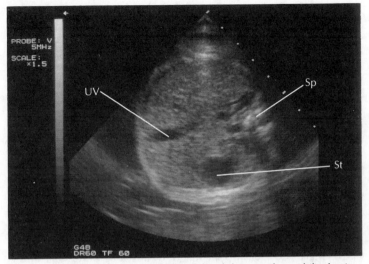

Fig 4.7 A section through the middle of the abdomen. The umbilical vein (UV) is visible on its way from the cord to the heart (St=stomach, Sp=spine).

assessed by the presence of urine in the baby's bladder and the amount of amniotic fluid, most of which comes from the baby's urine. In the absence of amniotic fluid around the baby prior to birth, there is often inadequate lung development. This is a common cause of death of babies with poor kidney function before birth.

Kidney abnormalities occur in approximately 0.8 per cent of babies. These include absence of one or both kidneys, cysts and blockage of the outflow of urine. Some of these abnormalities result in the death of the baby either before birth or immediately after. Those babies with a blockage of the outflow below the level of the kidneys may occasionally be suitable for treatment by inserting a tube above the level of the blockage to drain into the amniotic space (see Chapter 10).

**Hydronephroses** are fluid collections within the baby's kidneys prior to birth. If the amount is very small then it is of no significance to the baby's development. If the amount is large then it may be due to a blockage somewhere in the outflow from the kidneys. If the amount of fluid is intermediate in volume, it may be suggested that the baby be reviewed at intervals during pregnancy to ensure that the volume does not increase. The majority of these babies are delivered at the due time and are perfectly healthy. An ultrasound examination may be performed on the baby after birth to check how much fluid remains in the kidney. The unknown factor with these small fluid collections is whether they could be caused by urine flowing back up to the kidney from the baby's bladder when it passes urine. If this is discovered later in childhood, it can be readily treated.

# ▌ LIMBS

During an examination of the baby each of the limbs is inspected. As calcium starts to form in the bones by the end of the third month of pregnancy, they stand out as dense white lines. The soft tissues, such as muscles, are seen around the bone in figure 4.8. It is usually a simple matter to measure the length of any long bone, that of the thigh (femur) being the commonest.

**Dwarfism** is diagnosed if the length of the bones in the limbs is below the normal range. The diagnosis may be made as early as 14 to 16 weeks, but may not be possible until as late as 22 weeks. The limbs of babies affected by dwarfism increasingly fall below the normal range as pregnancy advances. While some babies with dwarfism, although short, lead a normal life, there are a large number who also have abnormalities in other regions of the body. In such cases, the baby may not survive after birth. Bone fractures may occur prior to birth in conditions such as **osteogenesis imperfecta** (brittle bones). In this condition the bones break very easily and may be markedly bent prior to birth.

# ▌ FEET AND HANDS

The baby's feet are readily seen on ultrasound and may be checked to ensure that the foot is at the appropriate angle to the lower part of the leg. Club feet, if severe, may be detected prior to birth as the foot is twisted around on the lower leg.

Figure 4.9 shows the hands and fingers. Sometimes it is easy to count the fingers but depending upon the position of the hand it may

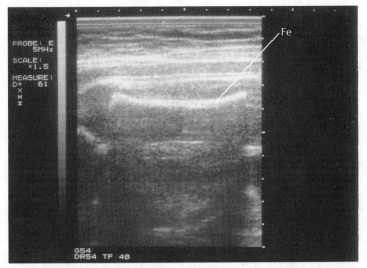

Fig 4.8 A section along the length of the thigh showing the femur (Fe), the bone within it.

Fig 4.9 The hand, with five fingers clearly seen.

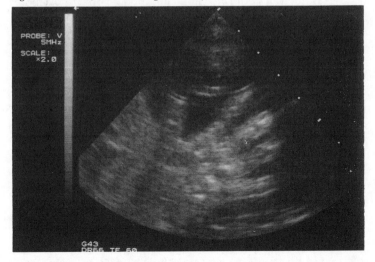

also be very difficult. Therefore, extra or missing fingers may at times be difficult to see. In addition, abnormalities in the shape of the hand or position of the fingers are occasionally detected.

# ▌UMBILICAL CORD

The umbilical cord is seen in figure 4.10 as a chain-like structure. If a section is taken across the cord the three vessels may be seen within it. Pregnant women often ask if it is possible to see the cord around the baby's neck. This can be seen, but it is very common and rarely causes any complication. It is likely to be associated with difficulties at delivery only if it wrapped tightly around the neck several times.

# ▌Errors and Pseudo-errors

Ultrasound cannot detect all abnormalities in all babies. Anybody can make errors and this certainly happens with ultrasound. Simply because there is a complication of pregnancy does not mean that it should have been diagnosed by ultrasound. Before you accept that ultrasound 'missed' a complication, consider each of the following factors:

(i)    Was the scan performed at an appropriate time to diagnose that complication? For example, in the first three months of pregnancy few abnormalities can be detected. Even late in pregnancy one or two limbs or the baby's spine may be virtually impossible to see properly.

(ii)   Because an abnormality is severe, it is not necessarily readily detected. A port-wine stain on the face may be unsightly but would not be detectable on ultrasound. As mentioned above, most babies with Down syndrome may also be missed.

(iii)  The position of the baby at the time of the scan affects the ability to detect abnormalities. If it is lying face up, the spine may be difficult to see properly but the face and chest are likely to be clearly visible. If it is lying face down, the heart and face may be masked but beautiful views of the spine obtained. The baby will often turn during the scan so that all of it may be seen well, but this does not always happen.

(iv)   An abnormality might be seen but the cause of it misinterpreted. A cyst in the abdomen may be part of the bowel, in which case it is usually of no consequence to the baby, or it

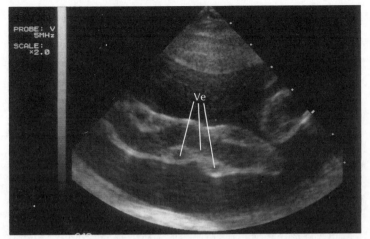

Fig 4.10 The umbilical cord showing the three blood vessels (Ve) within it.

      may be blocked kidneys with the most dire consequences.
(v)   Expectations as to what may be detected at your scan depend
      on the equipment used, the skill of the doctor and the build of
      the woman having the scan. It is much harder to see clearly if
      the woman is obese or has surgical scars on the abdomen.

# ▌ OVER-DIAGNOSIS

Over-diagnosis can be as important as under-diagnosis. The anxiety
suffered by parents who are told that their baby has a problem, no
matter how minor, only to find out later that it is normal, cannot be
overestimated. For example, one well-recognized abnormality diagnosed is fluid on the kidney — hydronephrosis. Many a pregnant
woman has been told her baby has a hydronephrosis when it is only
a small, normal amount of fluid in the kidney's collecting system
which later disappears without treatment.

In the first three months of pregnancy it is also normal for the
skin of the abdomen to be open with the intestines developing outside. If noted then, this should not be called an abnormality as the
intestines later return into the abdomen. If the finding is present at
four months, however, it is undoubtedly abnormal.

A low-lying placenta early in pregnancy can also cause a false alarm. Couples have been known to cancel overseas trips because the placenta looked low on ultrasound only to find later that it was normal and did not prove to be a problem.

# ▌Questions

## CAN I TRUST MY DOCTOR TO TELL ME EVERYTHING?
Doctors today usually believe in telling their patients about any complication of pregnancy. If you are concerned that you are not being given the full story, then ask, but important facts are rarely kept from pregnant women. It is possible you will not receive the results of your scan on the day it is actually performed. Technicians are often restricted in the information they can give to patients and are usually not permitted to counsel them. There is never any problem in asking in advance whether you will receive complete information at the time of your scan or whether you will have to wait until you return to your obstetrician.

## WHY CAN'T I SEE AS MUCH OF THE BABY AS I COULD EARLY IN PREGNANCY?
Strangely, you will find it harder to make out the features of your baby later in pregnancy than you could in the early stages. The baby becomes too large to fit readily on the ultrasound screen and is less likely to lie in a position that allows a life-like profile view to be obtained.

## WHAT ABNORMALITIES CAN YOU DETECT?
In a book such as this it is impossible to list all the abnormalities that may be detected in your baby. The general principle is that every time you see a normal structure then some abnormalities are excluded. This chapter gives you an idea of some of the more common abnormalities which can be found.

## CAN YOU COUNT THE FINGERS AND TOES?
Yes, these can be counted but it may be difficult. If you have previously had a baby who had extra fingers and toes, particularly if these were associated with other abnormalities, then it is appropriate to spend a long time counting. It is not practical to count all the fingers and toes of every baby.

# 5 CAUSES OF ABNORMALITY IN BABIES

If you wish to make a fully informed decision about tests for your baby then you need an overall understanding of the causes of abnormalities. There is a tendency to believe that the only important ones are Down syndrome and spina bifida. While these are important causes of major handicap, they are just two of an array of mostly rare conditions a newborn baby can have. In this chapter we will look at the wider picture of genetic abnormalities, what causes them, how common they are, and which can be detected before birth. Chapter 4 covered those that can be detected by ultrasound while the next two chapters will look at two more techniques — amniocentesis and chorionic villus sampling (CVS).

## The Chromosomes and Genes

Before looking at specific abnormalities, it is important to have some understanding about the chromosomes and genes. Cells of the baby collected during procedures such as amniocentesis and CVS are most often tested for chromosome and single gene abnormalities.

Humans have about 50 000 pairs of genes or inherited characteristics which are contained within 23 pairs of chromosomes, one in each pair received from each parent (see figure 5.1). The same chromosomes, and genes they carry, are present in every cell of the body. One chromosome pair determines the sex of the individual; females have two X chromosomes and males an X and Y. The remaining 22 pairs are called autosomes and along with genes on

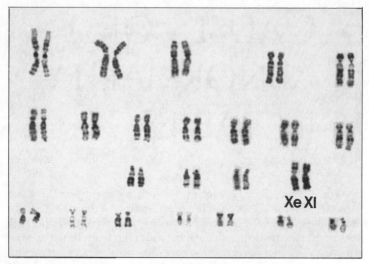

Fig 5.1 A normal chromosome analysis of 46 chromosomes.

the X chromosome determine the many characteristics of each human being such as hair and skin colour, appearance, height and intelligence. Individual chromosomes contain hundreds of genes as shown on figure 5.2, each of which represents in chemical code the information to allow the body to make one specific protein with a unique function. Each gene is located at a specific position on its chromosome and can be found at the same place in all people.

## ∎ Testing a Baby's Chromosomes before Birth

Both the cells that float in the amniotic fluid and those in the placenta are derived from the baby. They have the same chromosome make-up as the baby so can be sampled for analysis. As only a few cells are shed into the amniotic fluid a relatively large volume (around 15 ml) needs to be taken to reliably find enough cells for chromosome analysis. This method is known as amniocentesis. Chorionic villus sampling (CVS) involves the analysis of cells from the developing placenta or chorion. The baby's blood is occasionally sampled from the umbilical cord or heart when there is doubt about

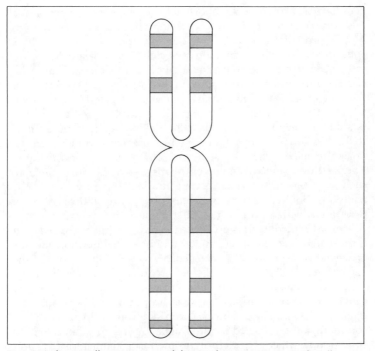

Fig 5.2  A diagram illustrating one of the 46 chromosomes in each cell.
Each of the shaded areas is a gene which may be responsible for one
characteristic. Often several genes are responsible for determining a single
characteristic such as hair colour, colour of eyes, baldness etc.

the results of amniocentesis or if there is a need for quick results.
Specimens can be taken from other parts of the baby's body such as
urine, but this is rare.

# ▌Can all Abnormalities be detected before Birth?

It is estimated that about 4 per cent of liveborn babies have an
abnormality, the cause of which is unknown in most. About 0.6 per

cent have a chromosomal abnormality, 1 per cent have one of the 5000 or so rare single gene disorders and at least 2 per cent are born with a structural malformation. The latter are disorders such as spina bifida, heart malformations and cleft lip and palate, which are influenced by genes as well as unknown other factors. It is only the chromosome abnormalities, some of the single gene disorders and a few congenital malformations which can be detected by amniocentesis or CVS. As these make up only a small percentage of the possible problems, it is clear that the tests do not guarantee a normal baby. This is an important point because many women regard a normal result on the tests as a stamp of normality on the baby. There are other more common problems associated with pregnancy such as prematurity, which occurs in about one in 20 births. In addition, about 10 per cent of babies grow poorly in the last half of pregnancy, with increased risk of complications occurring.

**Mental retardation** is probably the most feared abnormality. It is estimated that about one in 200 (0.5 per cent) newborn infants are severely or profoundly retarded. Many die early so that by the age of five, 0.3–0.4 per cent of children are intellectually impaired. Estimates vary on the contribution of causes. At the most, 40 per cent of mental retardation is due to a chromosome abnormality and might be detected before birth. Down syndrome is by far the most common cause, followed by the fragile X syndrome, an inherited condition in which the X chromosome has a characteristic abnormality when seen through a microscope. Most of the remaining 60 per cent of mentally retarded infants cannot be detected prior to birth. Some are the result of single gene disorders, others are the result of external factors such as maternal infection or lack of oxygen before birth. At least a third of cases have no known cause.

With current rapid advances in medical genetics, the range of disorders amenable to prenatal diagnosis is likely to widen rapidly. It has only been possible in the last few years, for example, to diagnose haemophilia and cystic fibrosis prenatally. Currently, about 250 single gene defects can be detected but not everyone can be screened for all the disorders for which tests exist — there are simply too many tests. Unless your baby is at special risk of a particular disorder, invasive testing will only tell you whether your baby's chromosomes are normal and its sex. Amniocentesis will also show whether there is a risk of spina bifida. If your baby has any other abnormality, such as a new mutation, it would not be detected unless visible on ultrasound.

On the brighter side, of the 4 per cent of babies born with an abnormality, about half are not serious and include such conditions as a port wine stain or an extra toe. In the best hands, ultrasound is likely to detect an abnormality in up to 1 per cent of babies, particularly many of the more serious conditions.

# Single Gene Defects

There are about 5000 recognized single gene defects, most very rare conditions, inherited from generation to generation. In the past, it has been difficult to diagnose such conditions prior to birth, even if a couple had a previously affected child, because the fault may lie in one specific gene. The first to be diagnosed before birth were those conditions such as metabolic disorders which produce an abnormal substance that can be detected in the amniotic fluid or baby's blood.

The most recent major development in diagnosis is by direct analysis of DNA, the building blocks of chromosomes. Scientists throughout the world are now attempting to determine the actual site on the chromosome where each of the genes occur. As knowledge of the location of genes increases, some diseases which occur because of abnormalities in either one or small numbers of genes can be diagnosed by studying the chromosome itself. Some are detected by probes for the actual gene, but more often it is nearby marker genes that are tested.

Analysis is not normally carried out unless there is a history of a disorder in either the mother or father's family or the couple already has an affected child. In such cases, a geneticist will be able to tell you the chance of a defective gene being passed on to your baby and whether it is likely to cause any major problems. This is because gene defects follow clearly defined patterns of inheritance, first outlined last century by an Austrian monk Gregor Mendel.

Put simply, each parent contributes a gene for a particular characteristic to each of their children. Normal genes and gene defects may be dominant or recessive. For dominant conditions such as Huntington's chorea, carriers of one copy of the gene defect will develop the disease. An affected parent will then have a one in two chance of passing it on to each of his or her children. Most conditions, however are recessive, and quite harmless to those who carry only one copy of the gene. For the disease to manifest, both parents must be carriers of the gene defect. The risk to each of their children is then one in four. Prenatal testing for those with a family history or a child afflicted with such disorders can be of profound assistance, and give them the courage to have a family.

While many single gene disorders produce seriously debilitating illnesses, they are also very rare, their incidence often showing wide regional variations. Some of the more common genetic diseases that can be diagnosed before birth are described below.

**Cystic fibrosis** is the most common single gene disorder amongst those of Northern European descent, affecting about one in 2000 liveborn babies. Cystic fibrosis is a condition that results in recurrent respiratory infections and is usually fatal in early adulthood. The recessive gene is carried by one in 20 people, upon whom it has no obvious impact. This condition could not be picked up before birth until it was discovered that abnormal enzymes were present in the amniotic fluid. This enzyme test had some problems, however, because of borderline results. Gene probes have now been developed which can give most parents a definitive result at CVS. Population screening may one day become available by testing everyone's blood so those couples at risk can be identified.

The red blood cell disorders known as **thalassaemias** cause major health problems in Italy, Greece, some of the Mediterranean islands and parts of South-East Asia. Gene probes can be used to test for the disorder in most at-risk families. For the rest, fetal blood sampling can be done at 18 weeks pregnancy to determine if the baby has inherited the gene defect from both parents. One copy of the gene has little impact while two copies result in severe anaemia and shortened lifespan.

Testing is also now available for **Huntington's chorea**, a dominant condition causing severe body movements plus mental deterioration after the age of 40. Those with relatives afflicted by the disease can be tested to find out if they will also develop it. Similarly, the condition can be diagnosed prenatally.

Haemophilia and Duchenne muscular dystrophy are **sex-linked conditions**, recessive gene disorders on the X chromosome, which are only likely to affect sons of women who are carriers. Each son will have a one in two chance of being born with the disease. Hae-mophilia is a bleeding disorder caused by the blood lacking a clotting factor. Usually couples with a high risk of a baby with haemophilia will be tested by CVS but some require fetal blood sampling at 18 weeks. Muscular dystrophy results in increasing muscular weakness, commencing in early childhood and usually resulting in death in early adulthood. This may also be diagnosed using CVS.

# ▌Chromosome Abnormalities

A chromosome abnormality may be so minor that it produces no ill effects in the offspring or so major that it results in miscarriage very early in the pregnancy. About half of all miscarriages are associated with chromosome abnormalities. There can also be a large range of major and minor developmental defects between these two ex-tremes. Those experienced at interpreting chromosomal abnor-malities can usually tell what if any, defect is usually associated with a particular chromosome abnormality.

The frequency of chromosome abnormalities at birth is about 6 per 1000. Of these, around one third result from rearrangements of chromosome material and the rest from variations in the number of chromosomes. Table 5.1 shows the more common chromosome abnormalities. Major abnormalities often result if there are more than the normal 46 chromosomes. Down syndrome, or Trisomy 21, in which there is an extra chromosome 21, is the most common chromosome abnormality to cause a major handicap in children (see figure 5.3). Another relatively common trisomy, or condition with an extra chromosome, is Trisomy 18. This is associated with a number of major abnormalities and usually results in the child dying shortly after birth. Triploidy, where there are three of every chro-mosome resulting in a total number of 69 chromosomes, usually results in a spontaneous miscarriage early in pregnancy.

Variations in the number of sex chromosomes make up about a third of the chromosome abnormalities found at birth. These are a range of conditions where the baby has either fewer sex chromos-omes than normal or extra copies of the X or Y chromosome. While these are possible to detect prenatally, sex chromosome variations present parents with some of the most difficult decisions.

TABLE 5.1 INCIDENCE OF SOME OF THE MORE IMPORTANT
ABNORMALITIES IN LIVEBORN BABIES

| Condition | Approx. incidence in 1000 births | Method of diagnosis | Proportion diagnosed |
|---|---|---|---|
| **Chromosomal** | | | |
| Down syndrome | 1.5 | Amnio/CVS | All |
| | | U/sound | Some |
| Turner syndrome | 0.2 | Amnio/CVS | All |
| | | U/sound | Some |
| XXX, XXY, XYY | 1.0 each | Amnio/CVS | All |
| **Single gene defects** | | | |
| Cystic fibrosis | 0.5 | CVS | All in some families |
| | | Amnio | Most |
| Sex-linked conditions e.g. haemophilia,* Duchenne muscular dystrophy (DMD) | 0.5 | CVS | All in some families |
| **Neural tube defects** | | | |
| Anencephaly | Varies | Amnio | All |
| | | U/sound | All |
| Spina bifida | Varies | Amnio | 98% |
| | | U/sound | Approx. 95% |
| **Others** | | | |
| Hydrocephaly | 0.5–3 | U/sound | Most, *after 20 weeks* |
| Cleft lip with or without palate | 1.4 | U/sound | Many, especially if severe |

| Condition | Approx. incidence in 1000 births | Method of diagnosis | Proportion diagnosed |
|---|---|---|---|
| Heart abnormality | 8 | U/sound | Approx. ⅓ including most of severe ones |
| Abdominal wall deficiency | 0.2 | U/sound | Nearly all |
| Kidney abnormalities | 8 | U/sound | Most, especially if severe |
| Dwarf | 0.2 | U/sound | Most, *after 20 weeks* |
| Club foot | 1.2 | U/sound | Many, especially if severe |

Note: 1) Approximately 4 per cent of live newborns have an abnormality.
2) Except where stated the ultrasound is assumed to have been carried out at 18–20 weeks.
* some families may need fetal blood sample for diagnosis.

Another quite common chromosomal variation found at testing is mosaicism. This is a term used when an individual has some cells in his or her body with one type of chromosomal make-up and other cells with another type. This individual then has some of the features derived from each chromosomal type, the final characteristics depending on the relative proportions of each. A child with mosaic Down syndrome has a mixture of normal cells and those with an extra chromosome 21. Such babies will have some of the features of Down syndrome but will be less severely affected. Chromosomal mosaicism is occasionally found in the placenta at CVS. It is usually associated with a normal baby with normal chromosomes.

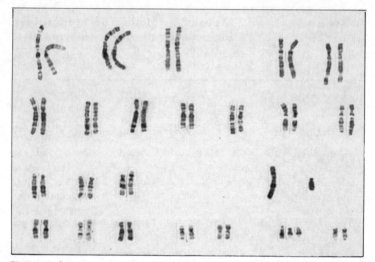

Fig 5.3  A chromosome analysis of a baby with Down syndrome — Trisomy 21.

# ∎ CHROMOSOMAL REARRANGEMENTS

These result from breakages in the chromosomes. Sometimes two chromosomes will have simply swapped pieces and the total amount of chromosome material will be normal. This is called a balanced translocation and usually has no effect on the child. At other times, chromosome material will be lost or gained as a result of a chromosome breakage. This situation is called an unbalanced chromosome translocation and is usually associated with mental retardation.

When an unbalanced translocation is found on amniocentesis or CVS, the baby is highly likely to be abnormal and most couples decide to terminate the pregnancy. If a balanced translocation is detected, the parents' chromosomes will be checked. Very often, one or other parent has the same balanced translocation and the baby can be expected to be healthy like the parent. If neither parent has the translocation there is a small chance that the child will be abnormal and a decision must be made whether or not to continue the pregnancy.

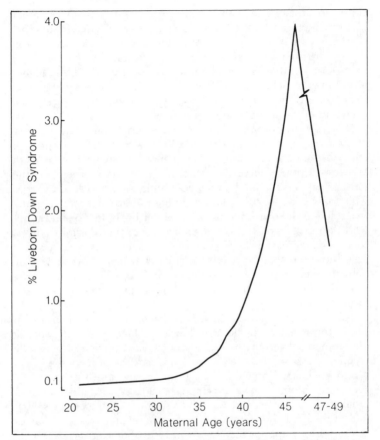

Fig 5.4 A graph showing the steep rise in incidence/likelihood of a Down syndrome baby with increasing maternal age over 35.

# ▌ DOWN SYNDROME

Down syndrome, previously called mongolism, is also known as Trisomy 21 because it is due to the individual carrying an extra chromosome number 21 in each cell. It is emphasized in antenatal diagnosis as it is the most frequent chromosomal abnormality resulting in a major handicap in a surviving infant. Many of the other abnormalities produce either minor defects or such major ones that the baby dies before or soon after birth. Babies with Down syndrome are mentally retarded and usually only reach an IQ of between 25 and 50, although with early education slightly higher scores may be achieved. They are also likely to have any of a number of other abnormalities, particularly of the heart structure which occurs in 40 per cent of affected babies.

Down syndrome occurs in 1 in 660 newborn babies. The majority of these occur 'out of the blue' to couples with no family history of chromosome abnormalities. The chance of having a baby with Down syndrome increases with the age of the mother, but the father's age has minimal influence (see figure 5.4). All of the eggs which a woman produces during her lifetime are present in a primitive stage in the ovaries at the time of her birth. It is believed that with the passage of years, and the ageing of these primitive eggs, there is an increased likelihood of chromosome abnormalities. It is important to realize that while the risk of having a Down syndrome baby increases with the mother's age, not all of the extra chromosomes 21 come from the mother. About a quarter come from the father.

Table 5.2 shows the chance of having a baby with Down syndrome at any particular age. The left column shows the chance of a woman delivering a live baby with Down syndrome. The middle column shows the chance the same woman has of having a Down syndrome baby detected if she has an amniocentesis at 16 weeks. The third column shows the chance of a baby with any chromosomal abnormality being detected at the time of amniocentesis. First look at the left-hand column and note that women of age 21 have a chance of only approximately one in 1600 of delivering a live baby with Down syndrome. By the time they reach 40 the risk has risen to about one in 110.

At first glance, one would imagine that most Down syndrome babies are born to older women but this is not the case. It is estimated that 35 per cent (or approximately one in three) of Down syndrome babies are born to mothers of age 35 or above. If a testing programme is used for women of 35 years and above then two thirds of the babies with Down syndrome would not be detected. This is because most women have their babies when they are young,

TABLE 5.2    RISKS OF CHROMOSOMAL ABNORMALITY

| Maternal age | Liveborn Down syndrome[1] | Amniocentesis[2] | |
| | | Down syndrome | All unbalanced chromosome abnormalities |
|---|---|---|---|
| | One in: | One in: | One in: |
| 21 | 1600 | | |
| 23 | 1300 | | |
| 25 | 1300 | | |
| 27 | 1100 | Amniocentesis figures not available | |
| 29 | 1000 | | |
| 31 | 900 | | |
| 33 | 600 | | |
| 35 | 380 | 260 | 110 |
| 36 | 290 | 200 | 95 |
| 37 | 230 | 160 | 80 |
| 38 | 180 | 120 | 65 |
| 39 | 140 | 100 | 55 |
| 40 | 110 | 75 | 45 |
| 41 | 80 | 60 | 34 |
| 42 | 65 | 45 | 27 |
| 43 | 50 | 35 | 22 |
| 44 | 40 | 30 | 19 |
| 45 | 30 | 20 | 15 |
| 46 | 25 | 17 | 12.5 |
| 47–9 | 60 | 45 | 18 |

*Sources:* [1] age 21–33, Hook et al 1988; age 35 up, Gardner & Sutherland 1989; [2] Ferguson-Smith & Yates 1984.

so even though individually they are at low risk, collectively they produce more Down syndrome babies.

When the results of data from amniocentesis were analysed it was a surprise to learn that the risk of finding a baby with Down syndrome at 16 weeks was greater than the chance of detecting it in a liveborn baby in a woman of the same age. The major reason for this difference is believed to be that babies with an abnormality have a much higher chance of dying prior to birth and therefore not appearing in liveborn figures. It is believed that approximately one in three Down syndrome babies who are alive at 16 weeks will die before, during or immediately after birth.

This factor presents a major difficulty in counselling couples of their chance of having a baby with Down syndrome. Which is the more important figure? Is it the chance of finding a Down syndrome baby at amniocentesis or CVS when the couple will have to decide whether to accept an abortion? Alternatively, is it more important to tell a couple the chances of them delivering a liveborn baby with Down syndrome whom they will then be responsible for? There is no uniformity on this complex question and couples are presented with both figures to analyse as they feel appropriate.

The last column in the table is the chance of a couple having a chromosome abnormality of significance detected at the time they have an amniocentesis. These include serious ones such as Trisomy 18 to less serious ones such as abnormalities of the sex chromosomes. Some would feel that this is the figure that should be presented to couples.

The table includes data from amniocentesis but not from CVS. These data were collected by a long-term collaborative amniocentesis study throughout Europe. The equivalent figures are slightly higher for results from CVS, as some of the live babies with a chromosomal abnormality at 10 weeks would die prior to 16 weeks so would not enter the amniocentesis figures. You will also notice that while information on liveborn babies is available down to 20 years of age, that on amniocentesis is not available below age 35. This is because amniocentesis has been offered on a regular basis only to women above this age.

For most couples the chance of producing a baby with Down syndrome depends entirely on the woman's age. If a couple has previously had a baby with Down syndrome, however, the chance of them having a second Down syndrome baby is increased. Under 35, the risk of recurrence is 1 in 200 for Down syndrome and a further 1 in 200 for other chromosome abnormalities, making 1 in 100 in all. Over 35, the risk is double the normal one associated with the specific age.

There is a rare type of Down syndrome, called the translocation Down syndrome, where the abnormality can run in families. As this is an uncommon problem we will not pursue it here. Its significance, however, is that the parents of a baby with this type of Down syndrome are always tested to see if they have a rearrangement of chromosomes that puts them at extra risk. If they do, other family members may be at greater risk too.

# ▐ SEX CHROMOSOME VARIATIONS

Sex chromosome variations make up about one third of the chromosome abnormalities and present parents with some of the most difficult decisions. This is because of the sometimes subtle abnormalities shown and the uncertain level of disability. Until the mid-1960s, knowledge about people with sex chromosome anomalies was based entirely on those who showed clinical symptoms, particularly intellectual handicap and disorders of behaviour. This provided a false view of sex chromosome abnormalities because only the most affected people were used to define the problems. Since then, large-scale screening of newborn infants has shown that 1 in 400 newborns has a sex chromosome variation and we now know that most will live relatively normal lives.

Newborn chromosome surveys began in the mid-1960s and continued over the next decade with the aim of finding out what kind of effect sex chromosome variations have on development. Some 307 children were identified and followed up in seven studies of consecutive livebirths in the United States, Canada, Denmark and Scotland. Girls with an extra X chromosome and boys with either an extra Y or X were found to be the most common, with an incidence each of about one in every 1000 births.

Girls with an extra X chromosome (47XXX) are taller on average and may have delayed puberty. Two thirds have normal intelligence while one third have borderline IQ or mental retardation. Boys with an extra X chromosome (47XXY), a condition known as Kleinfelter syndrome, are also tall. They have a mild reduction in intelligence but have frequent specific learning problems. They are infertile and have delayed or incomplete puberty which may be treated with hormones.

Boys with an extra Y chromosome (XYY syndrome) tend to be taller, are fertile, have normal intelligence and usually display normal behaviour. When the condition was first discovered, a higher incidence was found among prison inmates, leading to the conclusion that an extra Y chromosome predisposed carriers to aggressive and psychotic behaviour. Since then, follow-up studies have shown quite normal development in most, and the risk of behaviour problems seems to be lower than was first supposed.

A less common condition is Turner syndrome, the name given to the physical features of a girl with a missing X chromosome. The resultant sex chromosome pattern is called 45X. Turner syndrome occurs in about one in 5000 newborns. It is, however, much commoner in early pregnancy but most miscarry. Some Turner syndrome babies can be identified with ultrasound prior to birth. The features may include swelling of the tissues around the neck, fluid collection in other tissues, reduced amniotic fluid and poor growth of the baby. Such babies are very unlikely to survive until birth. When the baby is less severely affected, for example with minor swelling around the neck only, this may subside during pregnancy and the baby survive. If these features are detected with ultrasound, it is usual to check the baby's chromosomes. Only some will have Turner syndrome, others either having normal chromosomes or some other abnormality.

Babies with Turner syndrome who are born alive usually have less severe abnormalities. They may have webbing of the neck and an increased likelihood of heart and kidney abnormalities. While their intelligence is usually in the normal range, there may be some specific learning disabilities The child has small stature and does not have functioning ovaries, so she cannot usually have children, except by using a donated ovum and in vitro fertilization technology.

Because genetic testing only tells you about the chromosomes and not about the severity of any future disabilities, it can be quite confusing for parents considering what action to take. Although there have been large studies of children with sex chromosome variations, the range of possible outcomes is wide. The experiences of one couple who found out at amniocentesis that their baby boy had Kleinfelter syndrome, illustrate the dilemma.

The prognosis with Kleinfelter syndrome was not certain. Ben might simply be a tall, overweight, infertile person experiencing learning difficulties during middle childhood. Or he could be more severely intellectually disabled. He might develop secondary sexual characteristics only with the use of massive and continued doses of of hormones after puberty. But he might not. The literature suggested that he might have a predisposition to cancers of the testes or breasts. But it might not materialize. There was evidence of predisposition to psychotic illness. But he might be lucky. The information shifted and changed depending on what we read, the research methodology and whom we spoke to.

If your baby is found to have a sex chromosome variation, you should see a specialist geneticist. He or she will have the latest information on the condition. About half the couples with this finding decide to terminate the pregnancy. Your decision will be based on your own family circumstances and expectations.

# ▌Neural Tube Defects (NTD)

Neural tube defects are malformations of the baby's nervous system which have a strong genetic component but the precise mode of inheritance is unknown. Inheritance of NTD is described as multifactorial — that is it depends on a number of genes as well as external influences. Recent studies have suggested it may be related to low maternal vitamin levels at critical stages in the development of the baby, but this is still being investigated.

The incidence of neural tube defects varies throughout the world, the highest being in Northern Ireland where one in 120 babies are affected. In Australia and the United States, it affects about one in 500, while in Japan the incidence is less than one in 1000. If a couple have had a previous baby affected with a NTD or have the condition themselves, the risk of it recurring in each subsequent pregnancy rises to about one in 30. If they do have a recurrence, the chances of it being either a spina bifida or anencephalic will be equal. **The incidence of NTD is not related to the age of the mother.**

There are two main types of neural tube defect: **anencephaly**, in which the skull and brain do not form properly, and **spina bifida**, in which part of the spinal column is open. Babies with anencephaly are stillborn or die shortly after birth because most of the brain is missing, while the problems caused by spina bifida depend on the size of the opening, its location and the amount of damage to the spinal cord and brain. If the defect is small, low in the spine and covered by skin, there may be no problems or mild difficulties with leg weakness and poor sensation. More often, the defect is large and not covered by skin. The spinal cord and its membranes may protrude through the opening and lie in a sac on the baby's back. This often ruptures during pregnancy or at the time of delivery. The nerves to the lower part of the body, the legs, bladder and the bowel, pass through the defect. If they are damaged, there is a variable degree of paralysis of the legs and loss of control of the bladder and bowel.

Babies with spina bifida also develop fluid on the brain (hydrocephaly) because they have an associated blockage to the flow of fluid from the brain. Varying degrees of mental retardation may occur, preventable in some cases by draining excess fluid through a shunt. Children with severe spina bifida may have a short lifespan. Some may be suitable for surgery to close the defect in the back. This protects against infection, but will not restore lost function.

# ▍ TESTS FOR SPINA BIFIDA

Assessing the level of a substance known as alpha-fetoprotein (AFP) in the amniotic fluid surrounding the baby was the first test developed for spina bifida. This is raised in about 98 per cent of affected babies. AFP is produced by babies prior to birth and is present in their blood stream and spinal fluid. The level peaks at 13 weeks then decreases slowly until 40 weeks. If there is a defect in the skin, there will be a marked increase in the level of AFP that crosses to the amniotic fluid and mother's blood. Women having an amniocentesis in the first half of pregnancy are routinely tested for AFP levels. In some places all pregnant women are offered a test for AFP in their own bloodstream. This is discussed in Chapter 9.

Another test which can also be carried out on amniotic fluid is for acetyl cholinesterase. When levels of this enzyme are also raised, it provides extra confirmation of an abnormality. CVS cannot be used to diagnose neural tube defects.

# ▍ ULTRASOUND DIAGNOSIS OF NTD

Until recently all couples with a past history of spina bifida or anencephaly and those with an unexplained elevation of maternal serum AFP were offered amniocentesis. With increasing sophistication of ultrasound equipment this is now not always performed. After 16 weeks, ultrasound will diagnose about 95 per cent of spina bifida cases and all cases of anencephaly. A couple who have had a previous baby with spina bifida have a 1.5 per cent chance of anencephaly — all of which will be detected by ultrasound — and a 1.5 per cent chance of spina bifida. If the spine and head appear normal on ultrasound, the risk of spina bifida falls to one in 1300. If the ultrasound is performed by an experienced operator who is able to obtain good views of the baby's head and spine, there is a reasonable case for not proceeding with amniocentesis. Additional reassurance can come from a normal maternal serum AFP result if this test is available.

Apart from those with a previously affected baby, there are some other pregnant women who have a slightly higher than normal risk. These include parents who have a near relative with spina bifida, and those on some medication e.g. epileptics who are controlled on certain drugs. Many such couples have a risk of approximately one per cent of a baby with spina bifida in any pregnancy. Using the same logic as above, a normal ultrasound will be incorrect in only one in 5000 births. Ultrasound alone is therefore usually used for such couples together with a maternal serum AFP test if available.

# Genetic counselling

Counselling about genetic diseases is available at several levels. It is generally your obstetrician who will discuss any appropriate prenatal tests with you. He or she will be able to tell you what increased risks you run because of your age or other factors, and indicate what tests are available, their risks and where expertise is available to have such tests. Some diagnostic centres offer formal genetic counselling sessions to all women considering testing. It is important that some form of information, be it written or verbal, and be it provided by your obstetrician or counsellor, be available before you make any decisions.

Counselling sessions typically last about 30 minutes to an hour. More than two thirds of couples seen for counselling are recommended because of advanced maternal age. These sessions will cover the chromosomes, the differences between amniocentesis and CVS, the risks of miscarriage from the procedures and the risks of having a Down syndrome baby. The counsellor will explain the condition so that the woman has a full understanding of what her options are. Common misconceptions will also be cleared up such as the idea that you are at lower risk because you are healthy or that bleeding in early pregnancy is a contra-indication to testing.

Another routine part of genetic counselling is the recording of a short family history. This is to make sure there are no other relevant inherited problems within either parent's family. For those having counselling for reasons other than advanced maternal age, such as the presence of a rarer genetic disorder, family histories are very important. The counsellor will need information about any illnesses affecting your parents, their brothers and sisters, as well as your brothers and sisters and their children. If any previous pregnancies led to miscarriage or loss of the baby at birth or early in life, information will be needed about the cause or the name of a doctor who may be able to provide details. The counsellor will help determine what extra risks you, as a couple, have of producing a child with a specific genetic disease, and what this disease would mean for the child if affected.

Such discussions will also be able to alleviate fears a woman might have about the impact of drugs taken before she realized she was pregnant. There is no evidence to indicate an increased birth defect risk with the most commonly used medications.

After counselling, some women — particularly those who have suffered from infertility problems — are not prepared to place their pregnancy at any risk and decide not to go ahead with testing. Other couples are adamant about not bringing an abnormal baby into the world. Nearly all women make the decision beforehand that they will terminate a pregnancy if the baby has Down syndrome. It is important that everyone undergoing testing has a full understanding of what that will involve. With amniocentesis, for example, a termination is done at 18–20 weeks, usually by inducing labour, although in some centres it may be carried out surgically through the cervix by dilation and curettage.

# ▌ Summary of Reasons for Testing

You are likely to be referred for an amniocentesis or CVS if you fall within any of the following categories:

(i)     Advanced maternal age is the major reason for testing, accounting for at least two-thirds of women referred. The precise minimum age at which women are offered tests varies from 35 to 37 years, sometimes taken at the date of the procedure and others times from the expected time of delivery. The age that is chosen depends on available local resources and the opinion of local experts. The flexibility of this 'minimum age' requirement also varies.

(ii)    A couple with a past history of a baby with a chromosome abnormality.

(iii)   A parent with a chromosome abnormality.

(iv)    A woman who has had three or more miscarriages.

(v)     Subtle ultrasound findings which may mean there is an increased chance of a baby having a chromosome abnormality (see Chapter 4).

(vi)    Other ultrasound indications — these include significant structural abnormalities of the baby, major reductions in its growth and abnormalities of amniotic fluid volume.

(vii)   Abnormal results from biochemical tests on the mother — this includes an abnormal level of AFP in the mother's blood and other such tests as discussed in chapter 9.

(viii)  Some couples at high risk of having a baby with a neural tube defect, especially those who have previously had a baby with anencephaly or spina bifida and those with a raised maternal serum AFP.

(ix)    Those couples with a single gene disorder such as muscular dystrophy, haemophilia or thalassaemia in the family.

# ▌Questions

## I HAVE A CLOSE RELATIVE (E.G. SISTER, BROTHER, COUSIN) WITH DOWN SYNDROME. WHAT ARE MY CHANCES OF HAVING SUCH A BABY?    Your chances of having a baby with Down syndrome are not increased above those of any other mother of your age. In the unusual circumstance of the affected person having the rare translocation type of Down syndrome, the parents and other normal family members may have a chromosome rearrangement which increases their risk. It is likely

that the parents of the affected person will know if this is the case.

## I AM YOUNG BUT AM VERY WORRIED ABOUT A FETAL ABNORMALITY. MAY I HAVE AN AMNIOCENTESIS OR CVS?
It is important if you are in this situation that you look closely at why you wish to have the test done and what you would do if the test did show an abnormality. You will need to enquire whether amniocentesis is available to people like yourself. Some centres have limited resources and offer these relatively expensive tests only to couples who fit within certain guidelines.

## EARLY IN PREGNANCY I DRANK TOO MUCH ALCOHOL/TOOK DRUGS/HAD AN X-RAY/HAD A SEVERE ILLNESS; SHOULD I HAVE AN AMNIOCENTESIS OR CVS TO CHECK MY BABY
None of these external factors increases your chance of having a baby with a chromosomal abnormality. It may be appropriate with some of them to have a careful ultrasound at 18 to 20 weeks but amniocentesis does not test for damage by any of these substances.

## WHO MAKES THE DECISION AS TO WHETHER AMNIOCENTESIS OR CVS IS BEST FOR ME?
The decision is yours. In this book we have attempted to provide information to allow you to make your own decision. Chapters 6 and 7, which detail the differences between the two tests, should help you decide which is most suited to your situation. Your obstetrician plus local counselling services are also available to help you.

# 6 AMNIOCENTESIS

Amniocentesis (pronounced amneo-sen-tee-sis) is the withdrawal of a sample of fluid from around the developing baby. It involves passing a needle through the skin of the mother, the wall of the uterus and on into the sac containing the amniotic fluid (see figure 6.1). This test can be carried out at any stage of pregnancy although it is most commonly done at around 16 weeks.

## Development of the Test

Amniocentesis was the first test introduced in which a needle was used to invade the environment of the developing baby. It was first carried out in the 1930s to inject dye into the uterus to help outline the baby on X-ray. By the 1950s it was also used for testing a baby whose blood group was incompatible with its mother's. Amniocentesis to test babies for genetic disease was first performed in 1967, and its use has escalated ever since. You can see, therefore, that it is only relatively recently that babies have been tested before birth and even more recently that the tests have been in widespread use.

Unlike other tests we will be discussing, amniocentesis was introduced before ultrasound was widely used. Without the benefit of ultrasound to help the doctor accurately place the needle, the method had a risk of one in 100 of causing a miscarriage. With the widespread use of ultrasound, many studies show this risk to have dropped to 1 in 200.

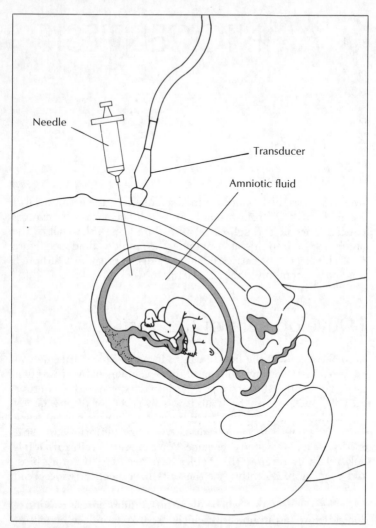

Needle

Transducer

Amniotic fluid

Fig 6.1 Amniocentesis: ultrasound is used to guide the needle into a pocket of fluid.

# ▮ Why have an Amniocentesis?

In general these tests are offered only to pregnant women who are at increased risk of producing a baby with very specific abnormalities such as Down syndrome. Amniocentesis is not regarded as a routine test available to every mother who wants to have all possible checks on her baby. This is because there is a small risk involved and because of the associated expense. For most young pregnant women the chance of having a baby with Down syndrome or other chromosome disorders is so low that the tests are considered unnecessarily risky. If these tests could pick up all abnormalities the situation might be different, but they can detect only specific abnormalities such as chromosomal defects. There are a host of rare genetic diseases that can be diagnosed by analysing the amniotic fluid, but most of these are only looked for if the parents have previously had a child with this disease.

The two most common reasons for undertaking amniocentesis are to check the baby's chromosomes and to look for spina bifida. In most centres older women, usually those 35 or 37 and above depending on local recommendations, are offered the option of amniocentesis or CVS. By this age the risk of miscarriage from the procedure is similar to that of having a baby with Down syndrome. In many ways, this is an artificial comparison because risks are perceived differently by different women, depending on their attitudes towards disabilities and their childbearing histories. Most Western countries now offer testing to those 35 and over, and sometimes to even younger women. Increasingly, however, all pregnant women are being offered a blood test at 16 weeks: hormones released from the placenta are tested (see Chapter 9) and if these show there is a higher than usual risk of Down syndrome, then amniocentesis is offered regardless of the mother's age.

Amniocentesis can be used to diagnose spina bifida, by measuring the alpha-fetoprotein (AFP) in the amniotic fluid. This is a cheap and easy test so it is routinely carried out on the amniotic sample even for those at low risk. Spina bifida is one of the few abnormalities which can be tested for by amniocentesis but not by CVS.

While most amniocenteses are carried out to look for genetic disease in your baby, occasionally it is done later in pregnancy for other reasons. These will be discussed in Chapter 10, and include testing a baby whose blood group is incompatible with that of its mother.

# ▌Timing of the Test

The usual time for performing amniocentesis is between 15 and 17 weeks. While women are keen to get the result as early as possible, studies on the risks when the technique is applied at an earlier stage of pregnancy, such as 10 weeks, are not yet complete. There was formerly another reason for preferring a later test. At 10 weeks there is only about 30 ml of amniotic fluid in the uterus which is smaller than the amount of water one can fit into a medicine glass but by 16 weeks about 200 ml is present, or six to seven times as much. This made it a much easier prospect for the doctor to place the needle into the fluid, allowing a smaller proportion of the total volume to be taken. Now with the aid of ultrasound, a needle can be put into the smallest volume of fluid. However, amniocentesis usually is still carried out at the traditional time until safety studies regarding the risk of 'early' amniocentesis are completed.

It is possible to do the test later than 17 weeks but the laboratory may take up to four weeks, and occasionally longer, to process it, which means the result comes back very late in pregnancy. Nobody wants to wait longer than necessary to get the results of a test on their baby. Sometimes it is unavoidable because a pregnant woman does not attend her doctor early in pregnancy, or the pregnancy is further advanced than expected. If you are unfortunate enough to have an abnormality detected on the amniocentesis and you want to have the pregnancy terminated, for both emotional and medical reasons this should be done as early as possible. The latest time an abortion can be performed depends on local laws and can be as early as 20 weeks or as late as 24 weeks, depending on which State and country you live in. If the baby has no prospect of survival, it is usually legal to perform an abortion at any stage.

# Termination of Pregnancy

From a medical viewpoint, abortion can now be carried out safely at any time of pregnancy. Local laws, however, restrict the stage at which it may be performed. One of the major disadvantages of amniocentesis is that if you choose to have an abortion following abnormal results the pregnancy will have advanced to 18 or 20 weeks, when it is usually necessary to induce labour. While complications are uncommon at any time, the risks are slightly higher at this late stage.

Uterine contractions are initiated by a substance called prostaglandin which may be injected into the amniotic fluid or up through the cervix around the membranes or simply placed in the vagina. It generally takes 12 to 24 hours until delivery, although most of this time is spent in waiting for contractions to start. During labour, pain relief can be achieved if necessary with Pethidine or an epidural anaesthetic. In some centres, late abortion is performed by dilation and curettage, a procedure similar to an early stage termination.

Even early in pregnancy it is a terribly difficult decision to have an abortion for a very much wanted baby, even though that baby is shown to have a major abnormality. If, however, that decision must be made at 20 weeks and you are already feeling the baby move then it is even harder (see Chapter 8 for a fuller discussion on this issue). There can be no denying that termination is likely to produce a very painful grief reaction. Women in this situation need plenty of family support and should be offered counselling.

# Preparation for Amniocentesis

You are likely to feel apprehensive and nervous prior to your amniocentesis, particularly if it is your first one. We hope to alleviate some of that fear by explaining the procedure and emphasizing that most women do not find it painful. It is an exciting experience seeing your baby on the ultrasound screen with all its human features. If you are able to relax enough to watch the TV monitor during the test you may find it fascinating. Many women find it helpful for their husband or a friend to attend amniocentesis with them. Your husband can see the ultrasound scan and provide moral support. If you both wish him to stay and watch the amniocentesis there is no reason why he should not do this.

You do not need to have any special preparation for amniocentesis. Your doctor may suggest you have an ultrasound examination sometime in the weeks before the amniocentesis if there is any doubt about how advanced your pregnancy is. In the past, women were required to have a full bladder for the ultrasound examination prior to amniocentesis. This is now no longer necessary, although your doctor might ask you to have some urine in your bladder. The ultrasound examination is done in the normal way, followed immediately by the amniocentesis without you having to move from the examination couch. There is no need to empty your bladder before amniocentesis.

Before you have the amniocentesis the doctor will want to know your blood group. This is because after amniocentesis, or any other tests involving passing a needle into the uterus, some blood cells from the baby may cross into your own circulation. If your blood group is a certain type, Rh negative, you will be given a special injection (anti-D) which destroys these cells — otherwise you might make antibodies yourself to destroy the baby's blood cells in your circulation. In your next pregnancy these antibodies could cross to that baby and destroy some of its blood cells. This is called Rhesus (Rh) disease, and although not a common complication of amniocentesis, it is one which is easily avoided with this injection of 'anti-D'. If, like 85 per cent of people, you are Rh positive you do not need this injection.

# Test Procedure

An area on the abdomen is prepared by cleansing the skin with antiseptic solution. A local anaesthetic would normally be available if you wish to have it. The ultrasound transducer is placed on the skin and moved around until an area is found where the needle can be inserted straight into the amniotic fluid without making contact with the baby or placenta (see figure 6.2). The needle is plunged rapidly through the skin, down to the appropriate depth (see figure 6.3).

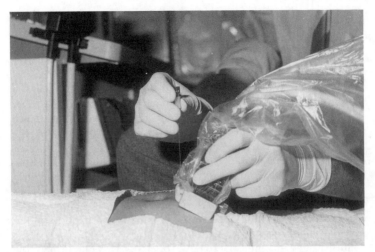

Fig 6.2 Amniocentesis: the fine needle is here being inserted through a frame to guide it to the correct place. The ultrasound transducer is in a sterile plastic bag.

Fig 6.3 Amniocentesis: The needle tip (Ne) is seen one third the way down the computer-generated line of the course of the needle (El=elbow H=head Pl=placenta).

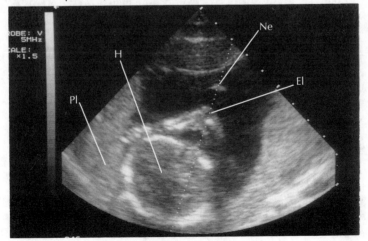

Most doctors watch the needle on the ultrasound screen from the moment it enters the skin until it is withdrawn, and so are able to adjust its position to avoid the baby if it comes near. There are two ways of guiding the needle. The first, shown in figure 6.2, involves passing the needle through a frame which is attached to the side of the ultrasound transducer. Those who use this method usually use the software of the ultrasound equipment to plot a dotted line down the screen and this is the course the needle will follow (see figure 6.3). It is then a fairly simple matter to line up the most readily available pool of amniotic fluid and place the needle into it to draw off the fluid. The alternative or 'freehand' technique is to hold the needle in one hand and the ultrasound transducer away from it in the other hand and watch the needle from a distance. Research has demonstrated no difference in the safety of the two techniques. The critical thing is that the operator be confident and experienced at that particular technique.

Surprisingly, it is unusual to have to pass the needle through the placenta to get into the amniotic fluid. Even when the placenta is on the front (or anterior) wall of the uterus it rarely covers the entire wall; a 'placenta-free' space is usually available somewhere. Occasionally there is no 'placenta-free' area. In this case the doctor would find a thin area of placenta and pass the needle accurately through this. Many doctors try to find a site high up in the uterus as this might help minimize the chance of fluid leakage after the test.

Once the needle is in the appropriate place a syringe is attached. The first 1 or 2 ml are usually discarded as they are more likely to contain cells collected from the mother's tissues. About 15 ml of fluid is withdrawn, then the needle removed and the heartbeat of the baby rechecked. If the test is carried out as described, there is virtually never any irregularity of the heartbeat afterwards.

The important point about the amniocentesis itself is that the doctor needs to be experienced in performing the technique under ultrasound guidance. It is reasonable to expect your doctor to be doing at least 50 amniocenteses per year.

# ▌Will the Test hurt?

Amniocentesis performed by an experienced doctor does not usually cause you more than mild discomfort. To many people it is no more painful than a blood test. When patients at a Melbourne clinic were asked to fill out a questionnaire after amniocentesis, 83 per cent said that the test was less painful than they had expected. Some 86 per cent said it caused no or only mild discomfort, while 14 per cent said it had caused some pain. Because most women dread the procedure, they are almost universally surprised that a needle can be passed into the uterus with minimal discomfort.

> I had read enough about amniocentesis to think that it would be awful. My husband came along and we had both built up a lot of apprehension. But I was lucky. The gynaecologist was terrific, probably the best around. It was definitely uncomfortable seeing the needle go into my stomach, but it was not painful. I'm very bad at reading maps and was distracted by the procedure, so the ultrasound had little impact. We had been ambivalent about having children, but my husband fell in love with our son when he saw him on the ultrasound screen.

For most women amniocentesis is a psychologically stressful experience, a focus for all their fears about abnormalities. As for physical pain, experiences vary. Apart from the skin and peritoneum, the needle passes through layers such as muscle, fatty tissue and the uterus which have few pain fibres. A very fine needle is used, usually 22 gauge which minimizes the risk and causes no distress to most women.

A local anaesthetic can be used to desensitize the skin, although most doctors do not encourage this. This is not just for the doctor's convenience but rather because the procedure is actually less painful if you do *not* have the local anaesthetic. The solution of local anaesthetic requires an injection which stings as it goes in and then a second needle must be inserted for amniocentesis. Experienced operators are able to pass the needle into the amniotic fluid on the first attempt on nearly every occasion. Most people will feel that the pain of the anaesthetic is worse than the passage of the needle without it.

# ▌After the Test

In previous years, patients were asked to stay in hospital after the test and have strict bed rest, but this is no longer considered necessary. After you have had the test it will probably be suggested that you sit down and wait for a short time before you depart. You will be quite capable of driving yourself home. Many women feel emotionally drained afterwards as they have been psychologically preparing for the test for some time and appreciate having somebody to accompany them home. It is probably a good idea to relax at home for the rest of the day, although there should be no reason to go to bed. Occasionally the needle may puncture a small blood vessel under your skin resulting in a bruise and minor discomfort. In general, most doctors would recommend a return to normal activities after the day of the test and for the remainder of the pregnancy.

# ▌Risks to the Baby

The most drastic complication and the one most universally feared is a miscarriage due to the amniocentesis. There have been many studies assessing the risks of the procedure and the most constant finding, one shown by virtually all, is that there is an increased risk of miscarriage. Putting a precise figure on that risk is more difficult. Different operators use different techniques which may have different complication rates. It is also difficult to tell if a pregnancy loss after amniocentesis is because of the procedure or whether it would have occurred anyway. It is likely that a miscarriage the day after was due to the test and one four weeks later not, but it is impossible to be sure. Figures are published which report the loss rates of major centres around the world. These estimate that amniocentesis increases the risk of miscarriage by about 0.5 per cent.

About 0.7 per cent of pregnancies which appear normal on ultrasound at 16 weeks will subsequently miscarry, if amniocentesis is not performed. This is called the 'background' rate. Unfortunately this background rate is not a precise figure. To find out how many pregnancies miscarry after amniocentesis, the background rate is subtracted from the total number who miscarry. This gives an approximate miscarriage rate due to the test which should be available information for potential patients.

One of the risks which you may be most fearful of is that the needle may penetrate your baby. Earlier studies showed that between one and three per cent of babies showed evidence after birth of being touched by the needle. Most cases involved dimples or skin scars. These mostly occurred prior to having modern ultra-sound machines to monitor the test. As the needle will be constantly watched with ultrasound on the television monitor, this can nearly always be avoided. Even if the baby comes near, the needle can be moved to keep out of its way. If the needle did touch your baby it would hurt as much as having a needle passed into the same place on your body, but little or no damage will result. Remember, babies have been tranfused before birth with needles passed into their legs and body at least a dozen times, without a single mark being visible on the skin after birth.

One large study suggested there was an increased chance of the baby being born with club feet or dislocated hips after amniocen-tesis. Other studies have not confirmed this. A group of children with these abnormalities was looked at and amniocentesis was not shown to be a cause. It is unlikely, therefore, that the risk of these postural abnormalities is increased by the test.

Several studies have suggested there is a slight increase of about 0.6 per cent in the risk of breathing disorders immediately after birth, particularly in babies born between 34 and 37 weeks. The reason for this increase is unknown. One suggestion is that it is related to the volume of fluid aspirated and that a maximum of 17 ml should be removed.

# ▌Other Complications

Complications rarely occur after the test. You may feel tired due to the anxiety associated with the procedure and its implications. Stu-dies of many patients suggest that amniotic fluid may leak from the vagina in about 1 per cent of amniocenteses, presumably leaking through a hole in the membranes. If this happened there would be a small gush of clear fluid from the vagina, usually in the few days immediately after the test. When this occurs at other times the out-look is very poor but after amniocentesis the leak usually lasts only a short time or is a single gush. The fluid loss usually settles rapidly and the pregnancy continues normally. Only rarely does the fluid loss continue.

If you have abdominal pain or if you lose water or blood through the vagina you should report it to your doctor — usually bed rest will be recommended. If this did happen you would notice without specifically watching for it. Any such symptoms usually settle. It does not necessarily mean you will miscarry.

The risks of the test to the mother are extremely low. Theoretically passing a 'foreign body', the needle, into the uterus could cause infection but this has rarely been reported. One study showed that generalized infection occurred in only one of 7579 patients.

# Minimizing the Complications

If a needle is passed straight into the amniotic fluid then there is very rarely blood staining — one series of 500 women were tested without a single specimen being blood-stained. Blood staining tends to occur if there are technical difficulties during amniocentesis. It has been suggested that if this happens then there is a two or three-fold increase in the risk of miscarriage, but even then the risk is quite low. Blood-stained amniotic fluid should not be confused with brown fluid. This is not due to the amniocentesis but usually to old blood which accumulated at the time of an earlier threatened miscarriage. When the amniotic fluid is brown there might be a slight increase in risk of miscarriage not because of the amniocentesis but because of the earlier bleeding.

Recent studies have shown that two insertions of the needle are required in 2–3 per cent of amniocenteses. It has been suggested that multiple needle insertions increase the miscarriage rate following the test, the risk increasing with each needle pass. Some studies have also suggested it may increase if the needle must pass through the placenta, although others have found no such increase. One would expect that the increased risk would depend on how thick a portion of the placenta was traversed. If care is taken to pass through a thin portion, the risk increase is likely to be minimal.

# Processing the Specimen

The specimen is sent to the laboratory where it is processed for analysis. It is put into a centrifuge which spins all the cells to the bottom of the flask. Some of the fluid is taken off the top to analyse for alpha-fetoprotein, the marker for spina bifida. The cells at the bottom of the flask are placed into a culture dish or bottle with culture medium containing antibiotics. This is then placed into an incubator and the cells allowed to grow. These cells come from the baby's skin, connective tissue, lining of respiratory, alimentary and urinary tracts and from the amniotic membranes.

The growth can take anything from a few days to occasionally as long as four weeks. When adequate numbers of colonies or cells have grown, the specimen is taken out of the incubator and carefully examined. At least fifteen cells are usually analysed. The chromosomes are counted to ensure that there are 46, and they are individually examined to make sure the structure or banding of each appears normal. This is a lengthy process requiring highly skilled personnel. A photograph is taken of the chromosomes from one or two cells. Each chromosome is then cut out, paired with its opposite member and placed in numerical sequence.

# ▌Waiting for the Results

The time taken for you to receive the results can be anything from one to four weeks or occasionally longer. These times vary because laboratory techniques differ. But even within one laboratory reporting times vary with the speed of growth of the cells and the workload. The wait for the result, is likely to be the most difficult part of the test for you. No matter how small the chance of your results being abnormal, your attention is likely to be focused on the result. The difficulty couples have coping with this delay until around 20 weeks pregnancy is the main reason CVS has become so popular (see Chapter 7).

# ▌Test Failure

Amniocentesis has now been refined to such a stage that once you have decided to have the test you can be almost sure it will be successful. However, even in the most experienced hands a test may fail and about 1 per cent of women require a repeat. This may happen either because fluid is not obtained or because of problems with the laboratory culture. Technical difficulties are uncommon during an amniocentesis, except in the rare situation when there is very little fluid around the baby. Occasionally, the laboratory may receive a good specimen but for some inexplicable reason none of the baby's cells grow so cannot be analysed. One reason for failed growth is that bacteria somehow get into the specimen. The laboratory also has difficulty if the the specimen is very blood-stained, a rare occurrence using the technique described.

# Amniocentesis in Multiple Pregnancies

If you have a twin pregnancy it is more likely they will be non-identical, particularly if you are over 35. In such a case, the risk of an abnormality in *each* of your babies is similar to that of a single baby. Therefore overall you have about double the risk of having a baby with an abnormality compared to someone with a single baby. If you have triplets the risk increases threefold and so on. Amniocentesis would still only be performed for the same reasons as a single pregnancy, such as advanced maternal age. Since two insertions of the needle are necessary with twins, there is likely to be an increased risk. Results vary but a recent report suggested the risk of miscarriage is around 1 per cent.

If amniocentesis is performed using the technique discussed in this chapter, then there is usually no problem sampling the fluid in the sac around each of the babies to test them individually. The doctor carefully searches for the membrane between the two babies and makes sure that fluid is taken from each sac in turn, usually by passing a needle through the skin at two separate sites. After taking the first specimen, a dye may be injected into the fluid, to ensure it is not sampled again. Many doctors believe this is no longer necessary.

If you plan to have an amniocentesis with a multiple pregnancy, it is worth considering what options would be available if a serious abnormality was found. Any abnormality would usually affect just one baby, with the other(s) being normal. In this situation three options would be available. First, you could continue the pregnancy knowing one is abnormal but being prepared to accept that outcome. Second, the pregnancy could be terminated, both the normal and the abnormal babies being aborted together. Finally, there is the option known as selective reduction, which involves injecting into the abnormal baby's heart a solution of a potassium salt, causing it to die instantly. This is a relatively new technique, and it has been difficult to interpret the data as to the risk to the surviving baby or babies, but it appears to be low. The dead twin stays in the uterus and is delivered at the end of the pregnancy without affecting the growth or wellbeing of the live baby.

Selective reduction would not be carried out if it appeared that the babies were monozygous (i.e. coming from one egg), because then there could be a mixing of the circulation of the two babies at the placenta in which case the death of one could affect the surviving identical twin. Fortunately, most twin pregnancies in which one of the babies is abnormal are dizygous (i.e. come from two eggs). If you would plan to accept option one, continuing with the pregnancy, then you might consider not having amniocentesis. Among those who believe it is best to take action if the result is bad, most opt for the injection rather than aborting the normal fetus as well.

# ▌ Questions

## HOW LONG DOES THE NEEDLE STAY INSIDE ME?
The time taken between insertion of the needle through the skin and removing it after withdrawing the fluid is around thirty seconds. Once the needle is placed in the fluid around the baby it does not have to be moved, so it does not hurt at all as the fluid is being withdrawn. You will have no 'pulling' inside and no other feelings as the fluid is removed from your uterus.

## CAN MY CELLS GROW IN THE LABORATORY INSTEAD OF THE BABY'S?   This is called 'contamination' of the specimen with your cells. As the methods described in this chapter are so reliable it is now very rare indeed for contamination to occur.

IF MISCARRIAGE OCCURRED, WHEN WOULD IT HAPPEN?   Unfortunately there is no simple answer to this question. There is no way of telling whether a miscarriage after amniocentesis is due to the amniocentesis or would have occurred anyway. Since miscarriages can occur at any stage in pregnancy whether or not you have an amniocentesis, there is no time that you can say you are 'totally safe'. It is presumed in general that miscarriages in the few weeks after amniocentesis are more likely to be due to the test than those that occur much later. The important thing to remember is that this is a low-risk technique and it is rare to miscarry as a result of it.

WHY IS THE FLUID YELLOW?   When red blood cells are broken down in the body a yellow substance called bilirubin is produced. The bilirubin tends to accumulate in the amniotic fluid in early pregnancy and gives it the yellow colour which is quite normal. As pregnancy advances the fluid tends to become clearer.

HOW DO YOU MAKE SURE THE NEEDLE WILL NOT TOUCH MY BABY?   At amniocentesis a pool of amniotic fluid is lined up well away from the baby and the needle placed straight into that fluid. While theoretically the doctor could go off course and touch the baby, or alternatively the baby could move into the path of the needle, as long as the doctor watches the needle with ultrasound, the baby is usually easily avoided. Even if the baby did come in contact with the needle, it would not be harmed, indeed, as we will see in Chapter 10 the baby is sometimes pricked by the needle deliberately for testing or treatment.

HOW MUCH FLUID DOES THE DOCTOR TAKE?   Usually about 15 ml which is less than 10 per cent of the amount of fluid present at 16 weeks.

HOW LONG DOES IT TAKE FOR THE FLUID TO BE REPLACED?   The baby continuously produces and removes the fluid around itself. By the end of pregnancy over one litre of amniotic fluid is produced daily by the baby and the same amount removed by it. It is hard to tell how long it takes for the total amount of fluid present to return to what it was before the amniocentesis, but it is presumably over the course of several days.

## WON'T THE FLUID LEAK OUT THE HOLE IN MY SKIN?
The needle used is so fine that the hole closes off immediately and fluid does not come out through the skin afterwards.

## I HAVE A BROTHER OR SISTER WITH SPINA BIFIDA. SHOULD I HAVE AN AMNIOCENTESIS?    Usually it is not
recommended. Your baby has approximately a 0.5 per cent risk of having spina bifida, with an equal risk of anencephaly. Ultrasound will detect all cases of anencephaly after 13 weeks and approximately 95 per cent of spina bifida at 18 weeks. If you have a normal ultrasound at 18 weeks then the chance of your baby having spina bifida is only about 1 in 2000. Amniocentesis would be unnecessarily risky by comparison. As an added precaution an AFP test on your blood may be suggested (see Chapter 9).

## CAN AMNIOCENTESIS TELL YOU THE BABY'S SEX?
Analaysis of the baby's chromosomes automatically indicates its sex. Your obstetrician can tell you the sex if you wish to know.

## IS IT TRUE THAT I MUST HAVE AN AMNIOCENTESIS IF I'M OVER THIRTY-SEVEN?    Amniocentesis is an option available to couples who are seeking prenatal diagnosis. There is never any compulsion to have the test. You are welcome to seek medical advice but ultimately you are free to make your own decision.

# 7 EARLIER TESTING WITH CVS

You may not have heard of chorionic villus sampling (usually abbreviated to CVS) because it is much newer than amniocentesis. It is, however, well beyond the research stage. Many centres have found a remarkably rapid swing away from amniocentesis to CVS, the great attraction being that the results are available very much earlier in pregnancy. There is, however, considered to be a greater risk of miscarriage with CVS. While only slightly higher than amniocentesis when performed by an experienced operator, the risk can range considerably. This chapter aims to tell you what to expect from a CVS test and to help you understand its benefits and risks.

Chorionic (pronounced ko-re-on-ik) villus sampling is a test involving the passage of a needle or cannula into the placenta in order to withdraw a few small fragments of the tissue into a syringe. It is called 'chorionic' because the chorion is the name for the placenta in the very early stages of pregnancy. The name 'villus' is derived from the microscopic appearance of the chorionic surface — large numbers of finger-like structures or 'villi' projecting outwards towards the lining of the uterus. Chorionic villus sampling is occasionally called 'placental biopsy' or 'placentocentesis'.

## Development of the Test

CVS was first used in Denmark in 1968 but was abandoned because it caused too many miscarriages. It was however quickly taken up by the Chinese who used CVS to determine the sex of some babies early in pregnancy to ensure that male children were born. It was first used to test for abnormalities in the USSR in 1982 and then subsequently in Europe. Initially, all specimens were taken by passing a cannula through the vagina and the cervix up into the uterus. But in 1984 the first successful attempts were made using the alternative approach whereby a needle is passed through the abdominal wall and uterus and then into the placenta.

When CVS was first used, many methods of obtaining placental tissue were tried. Success rates with these different methods varied but commonly they caused a very high miscarriage rate. As techniques were refined only those methods with a low miscarriage rate were used widely in clinical practice. Today all biopsies are taken under the guidance of ultrasound. In experienced hands, CVS is now believed to increase the miscarriage rate by about 1 per cent.

# ▌Why have a CVS?

CVS and amniocentesis are offered to pregnant women who are at increased risk of producing a baby with specific abnormalities. They are not general tests to see if the baby is normal. While there are a host of genetic diseases that can be tested for by analysing chorionic villi, most of the diseases are very rare and would only be looked for if there was a family history of a disorder which could be passed onto a child. There is only one common reason for testing chorionic villi, to check the baby's chromosomes. The reasons for performing CVS were discussed in detail in Chapter 5. By far the most common reason is because the mother is in her late thirties or forties and therefore is at greater risk of having a Down syndrome baby. The second most common reason is because a woman has previously had a baby with a chromosomal abnormality.

If the test is to be performed to check the baby's chromosomes there is a choice of CVS or amniocentesis. While most diseases which can be tested by amniocentesis can also be tested by CVS, there is one important abnormality for which CVS is not applicable — spina bifida.

There are two reasons why this inability to test for spina bifida on CVS is usually unimportant. Spina bifida is a rare condition in most

countries and unlike Down syndrome its incidence does not increase with the age of the mother. Therefore most women having a
CVS are at low risk of a baby with spina bifida. In addition, ultrasound is now so good at picking up spina bifida that it will usually be
detected if those women who have a CVS also have a scan at 18
weeks.

# Who should perform the CVS?

The best test for you depends on expertise in your region. Before
making your decision on amniocentesis or on transabdominal or
transcervical CVS (see below), you should ask your obstetrician
which techniques local experts usually perform. A major US study
suggested that approximately 75 CVSs need to be performed to
learn the technique. Performance improves considerably with experience. Independent follow-up of women who have undergone
CVS have shown miscarriage rates as high as 10 per cent. These high
rates can be attributed to the inexperience of the operators and
highlight the importance of selecting the best expertise available. It
has been suggested that skill improves over the first 100 cases of
transabdominal CVS and over the first 300 transcervical tests. To
maintain expertise at least 50 procedures per year should be performed. The doctor performing the CVS should also be able to tell
you how many patients miscarry after the procedure in his or her
particular practice. Experienced centres generally quote 1 per cent
as the miscarriage rate attributed to CVS. On top of this is the
'background' risk: even without the test about 2.5 per cent of
women whose pregnancy appears normal at 10 weeks will miscarry.
The background risk increases with the age of the pregnant
woman.

# When is the Best Time for a CVS?

The usual time to perform CVS is between 9 and 11 weeks. It can,
however, be performed any time during pregnancy. Tissue can be
obtained as early as 6 weeks after the last period but at this time the
chorion is spread very thinly around the whole of the developing
pregnancy sac; this would tend to make the test more difficult and
so probably more risky. By 9 weeks the placenta becomes thicker in

one area and it is possible to recognize where the fully formed placenta will be situated. This is an easier target for the needle.

If the direct method of chromosome analysis is used, it may provide the chromosome result in a few days. Otherwise, the laboratory needs between one and three weeks to process the specimen, in which case you will be told the result by about 13 weeks. At this time you do not look pregnant and have not felt movements. If you are unfortunate enough to have an abnormality detected and you request an abortion, it is still early enough to dilate the cervix and carry out a simple curettage operation. It takes only a few minutes and usually it is unnecessary to stay overnight in hospital. This technique can be used as late as 14 to 16 weeks and means that you need not go through labour. CVS can also be performed later in pregnancy when it is often called placental biopsy.

# Preparation for CVS

Your doctor may suggest you have an ultrasound examination some time before your CVS if there is any doubt about the age of your pregnancy or if you have had some complication such as bleeding. In addition, if a transcervical CVS is planned a swab may be taken from your cervix to look for bacterial infection to avoid the possibility of infection being introduced into the uterus at the time of CVS. Such an infection will usually be treated with antibiotics first or alternatively a transabdominal CVS performed instead.

You do not need to have any special preparation on the day of your CVS. The only thing your doctor may ask you to do is to have some urine in your bladder either for the ultrasound or for the CVS, particularly if it is transcervical. The ultrasound is carried out in the usual way, followed immediately by the CVS without you having to move from the examination couch.

As described in the previous chapter, the doctor will also want to know your blood group before CVS. This is because some blood cells from the baby may cross into your own circulation during the procedure. If you are one of the 15 per cent of mothers who are Rh negative, your body might produce antibodies to these cells which cause problems in subsequent pregnancies. Mothers in the Rh negative blood group will, therefore, be given an 'anti-D' injection to prevent such an occurrence.

# ▌How is the Test done?

There are three ways of passing a needle into the developing placenta.

(i)   The most widely used method has been to pass a cannula through the cervix and into the uterus to the developing placenta; this is transcervical CVS (figure 7.1).

(ii)  The second most commonly used method is to pass a fine needle through the skin of the abdominal wall, through the uterus and down into the placenta; this is a transabdominal CVS (figure 7.2). From the mother's point of view, this is very similar to an amniocentesis.

(iii) The final approach is to pass a needle into the vagina and then through the wall of the uterus into the developing placenta. This is similar to the first method, except that instead of being passed through the cervix, the needle is passed through the wall of the uterus and avoids the cervix. This method appears to be more invasive and so it is hardly ever used.

Which method is used depends partly on medical factors (see Table 7.1) but above all on the expertise of the operator.

## ▌TRANSCERVICAL CVS

For a transcervical CVS it is necessary for the bladder to be full. Prior to the test the doctor will check that there is an appropriate amount of urine in your bladder at the same time as the baby is scanned. You will then be asked to lie on your back with your legs lifted and held apart in stirrups at the foot of the couch. After washing in and around the vagina with an antiseptic solution the doctor passes a speculum (a metal or plastic object which holds the walls of the vagina apart) into the vagina to view the cervix. Having located the cervix, if necessary he or she grasps it with a pair of forceps. This may produce a pinching sensation.

The specimen is taken by passing a blunt cannula up through the cervix into the uterus, then advancing it into the developing placental tissue. By placing the ultrasound transducer onto the skin of your abdominal wall, the doctor is able to watch the cannula as it passes through the cervix and carefully guide it into the placenta.

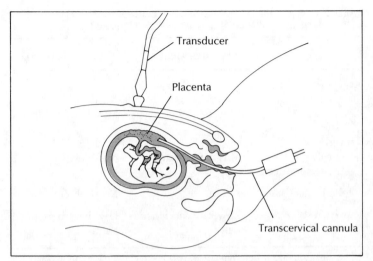

Fig 7.1 Chorionic villus sampling (CVS), using the transcervical method: a cannula is passed up through the cervix then guided into the placenta with ultrasound.

Fig 7.2 Chorionic villus sampling (CVS), using the transabdominal technique: a needle is passed through the abdomen down into the placenta.

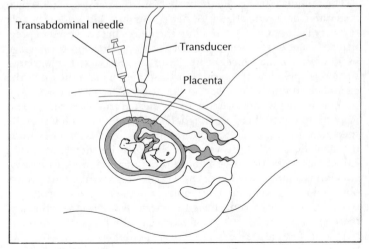

TABLE 7.1   FACTORS INFLUENCING THE CHOICE BETWEEN
TRANSABDOMINAL AND TRANSCERVICAL CVS

|  | **Transcervical** | **Transabdominal** |
|---|---|---|
| Access difficult: | | |
|   cervical fibroid | Difficult | No difficulty |
|   sharply retroverted uterus | May be difficult | May be difficult |
|   sharply anteverted uterus | May be difficult | No difficulty |
| Vaginal infection | Avoid | No problem |
| Risk of test* | Low in experienced hands | Low in experienced hands |

* The most important determinant of risk is the experience and expertise
  the doctor has of the test.

An anaesthetic is not used. Any irregularity of the wall of the uterus
can usually be negotiated by careful and gentle manipulation.

The cannula is made of either soft, bendable stainless steel, which
is sterilized between patients, or of a disposable plastic. Most people
feel very little as this is passed into the uterus because even in pregnancy the neck of the womb is sufficiently open to allow the passage
of this fine cannula. Once the tip of the cannula is into the placenta,
suction is applied to the syringe at the other end and the tip of the
cannula is moved around within the placenta to obtain tissue. The
cannula is then withdrawn, the tissue ejected from the syringe and
inspected to see if there is enough. If there is not enough villi in the
specimen, the test can be repeated by passing a second cannula
through the neck of the womb. Test repetition depends on the
experience of the operator and can occur in as few as 7 per cent of
cases and as many as 45 per cent. Usually if inadequate material is
obtained after two or three attempts then the procedure would be
rescheduled since by continuing to repeat the test on the same day,
there is an increased risk of miscarriage. The pregnancy and the
baby's heart beat are rechecked after the test.

Once the CVS has been completed, your legs are taken out of the stirrups and you lie on the couch for a short time before emptying your bladder. There may be some slight vaginal bleeding. It may be suggested that you sit and relax for a while before going home.

This test is not used if you have an untreated vaginal infection, are unable to accept any vaginal examination, have a fibroid low in the uterus which would be difficult to bypass, or if you present for CVS after 11 or 12 weeks.

# ▌ TRANSABDOMINAL CVS

If the transabdominal approach is used then most doctors would not ask you to have a full bladder. The ultrasound examination is carried out and instead of placing your legs into stirrups, you remain lying flat on the couch. The doctor then locates the best place to pass the needle through your skin and if local anaesthetic is to be used, injects it into that site. Most doctors give an anaesthetic, but it is difficult to know how much benefit it provides. It is used to anaesthetize the skin and the layers immediately beneath. It is not used to anaesthetize the layers deep inside the abdomen and if any discomfort occurs with this test, it is usually from these deeper layers.

The specimen is taken by passing a needle down through the wall of your abdomen as shown in figure 7.2 and into the placenta. This needle is carefully guided by watching it with ultrasound. It may be guided by using an attachment at the side of the ultrasound transducer to hold the needle on a predetermined course which is shown on the screen as a dotted line. An alternative technique is to hold the transducer at a distance from the needle to watch its advance. The best method to use is the one with which the operator is most comfortable.

Once the needle tip is placed through the wall of the uterus and situated in the placental tissue then the sample can be taken. This is usually done by feeding a second needle down the inside of the first and moving it up and down in the placental tissue whilst applying suction with a syringe at the other end. It can also be performed by applying suction to a single needle. The advantage of the two needle method is that if there is inadequate material then the fine needle can be painlessly passed down the inside of the wider bore needle to take a further sample. Depending on the width of the needle, it can take several aspirations to obtain enough material.

When the tissue has been inspected and found to be adequate, the needle is withdrawn. The laboratory likes to receive at least 10 mg for analysis. This amount of tissue is visible to the naked eye and looks like a few flecks floating in the fluid at the bottom of a flask. After the test, the pregnancy and the heart beat of the baby are checked before you leave the room.

Minor variations to the techniques described are used at different centres. A wide variety of needles are used, and indeed fine forceps may be used to take the sample of tissue rather than a needle. There are advantages and disadvantages of each technique but ultimately the equipment selected comes down to personal preference of the doctor. Even if you decide you would prefer a particular approach it is usually better to have whatever method is offered. If a doctor is asked to change his or her technique the results may not be as good. You are better to change to a doctor who uses the method you like rather than ask your own to change.

# Will the Test hurt?

For most women CVS is not a painful test. Whichever method is used it is readily tolerated. In the transcervical test, some people find having a full bladder and their legs in stirrups disturbing. If an instrument is used to grasp the cervix, it might cause some mild discomfort. Usually the passage of the cannula into the placenta is not particularly unpleasant.

If the CVS is transabdominal then it is usually tolerated well. It is little different to an amniocentesis and although a slightly wider needle is used, it is generally associated with little pain. In a survey of fifty women who underwent transabdominal CVS in a Melbourne practice, 90 per cent reported no or mild pain. The other 10 per cent described the pain as moderate and none reported severe pain. One situation that can cause considerable discomfort is in the rare case where the uterus is tilted backwards (retroverted) and the placenta inserted in the back wall of the uterus. This makes it more difficult to reach with the needle. Two women who have undergone CVS give their impressions of the procedure:

I had another surprise pregnancy and this time I chose a CVS. It was a new test and would only involve a curette rather than going through labour if a termination was necessary. From my reading, the risks weren't that much greater than amniocentesis. The procedure amazed me. The needle went through my abdomen, into the uterus and was dipped in and out. This had to be done four or five times, but it was not painful. I was quite philosophical about it. The pregnancy was unexpected and if it wasn't to be, then I would cope with that when the time came.

When I found out I was pregnant, I went to the gynaecologist quickly because I wanted to have a CVS. I had heard it was the same procedure as amniocentesis but that it was done earlier at 10 weeks. I found the risk of miscarriage of 1 per cent quite acceptable. Initially, my husband was against the test because he didn't want me to terminate the pregnancy if the baby was found to have Down syndrome. When I explained how a disabled child would reduce the amount of attention we could show our daughter, he mellowed. The actual test was frightening but straightforward. The needle only had to go in once and there was no pain, just discomfort. It was wonderful having test results back so early because it relieved all the pressures.

In the survey of fifty women who had transabdominal CVS seventeen (34 per cent) also developed abdominal discomfort after the test. This was described as mild by thirteen, moderate by three, and severe by one. The one woman with severe pain had a similarly severe reaction to having a blood test. The pain began between one and fifteen minutes after the CVS and lasted between two and twenty minutes. It was probably due to uterine contractions which subsided in all cases.

# ▌The Risk of Complications

The thought of passing a needle into the placenta with its very rich blood supply is initially frightening. Anybody who has seen the large blood vessels leading to the placenta would expect such a test to cause severe bleeding. Clinical trials have shown that this rarely happens.

As the needle does not enter the amniotic sac or pass near the baby there is very little chance of hurting the baby itself. The main risk is of miscarriage due to the test and experienced doctors who have performed large numbers of CVSs would usually quote it as around 1 per cent.

Complications of any procedure may be immediate or occur some time later. Significant immediate complications other than pain and failure to obtain a specimen are rare. It is possible to rupture the pregnancy sac at the time of the test but this is rare with an experienced operator. If this happens with a transcervical CVS the pregnancy may miscarry because the cannula leaves such a large hole. If on the other hand, it happens at transabdominal CVS it may not cause any complication as the needle is much finer. Another complication is the formation of a clot at the site from which the specimen was taken. Again this is rare and if it occurs it will usually resolve without any ill effect.

The most important delayed complication is miscarriage. This will not differ from miscarraige unrelated to CVS — both begin with bleeding. It is difficult to know the exact risk of CVS causing a miscarriage. It is estimated that if a baby is alive at 10 weeks there is a chance of about 2.5 per cent that it will miscarry anyway without being tested. The chance of miscarriage increases with the age of the pregnant woman. If she is 37 years or more then the figure rises.

To determine the risk of miscarriage due to CVS a study would need to be carried out in which women are randomly assigned to CVS or no test (not even amniocentesis later) and the miscarriage rates compared. This type of study is impossible as couples wish to have the right to choose to have a test if they are eligible. Two studies, one from Canada and one from the USA, compared the miscarriage rate after transcervical CVS to that after amniocentesis. They found that CVS caused 0.6 and 0.8 per cent more miscarriages than amniocentesis respectively. Both of these studies were carried out at multiple centres and some units produced better and some, worse results than this — emphasizing the point that the risks depend on who performs the test.

It should be noted that both studies included transcervical CVS only. Less information is available regarding the risk of transabdominal CVS, although there is some suggestion that it may be slightly lower. World figures in May 1990 of total pregnancy losses — the background rate plus those due to the test — were 3.2 per cent for 6850 women undergoing transabdominal CVS and 4.3 per cent for 18157 women given transcervical tests using a plastic (portex) cannula.

Significant complications other than miscarriages are rare following CVS. Some slight bleeding is common after transcervical CVS but rare after transabdominal. The bleeding usually settles within a few days. CVS should not damage the placenta. If the placenta is examined following CVS it is difficult to find any sign that the test was performed. There is no evidence of long term damage to the placenta — babies who have had CVS grow just as well as those who have not had the test.

Finally, there are reported cases of severe infection following transcervical CVS resulting in miscarriage and severe illness in the mother. Because of this, transcervical CVS is not carried out if there is untreated infection in the cervix. It is a very rare complication — no cases occurred in the 2235 women who underwent transcervical CVS in the USA study quoted above.

# ▌What to expect after the Test

After you have had the test it will probably be suggested that you wait for a short time before you go home. You will be quite capable of driving yourself home. However, many women feel emotionally drained afterwards as they have been psychologically preparing for the test for some time, and appreciate having someone to accompany them. It is probably a good idea to relax at home for the rest of the day, although there should be no reason to go to bed. While doctors may make slightly differing recommendations, the principles are that after any test in which a needle is passed into the uterus it is recommended that you rest at least the remainder of the day. In general, most doctors would recommend no restriction of activities the following day or for the rest of the pregnancy.

Some bleeding from the vagina is very common after a transcervical CVS. This bleeding often arises from the lower part of the uterus away from the pregnancy, either from the trauma to the uterus itself or from where the cervix was grasped. It usually settles very quickly but may be followed by some brown staining for a day or two as the last of the blood drains away.

Bleeding is rare after transabdominal CVS as the lower part of the uterus has not been interfered with. As discussed earlier some women have discomfort in the lower abdomen for a short time after the test. This nearly always settles very quickly and does not seem to be associated with a risk of miscarriage or damage to the developing pregnancy.

It is rare to have any other problems after a CVS. If you do have any other symptoms such as continued bleeding, pain or loss of fluid then it is important that you contact your obstetrician. Even if you are unlucky enough to have any of these symptoms they are likely to settle and your pregnancy continue unaffected.

If you do miscarry after the test, there is no way of telling whether the test was responsible as the symptoms are identical to those of any other miscarriage. The first thing you would notice is bleeding. Your doctor may then suggest you have an ultrasound examination to check whether the fetus is still alive. If it is alive then you should rest in bed until the bleeding stops. If you do miscarry it is not possible to predict when it will happen. Miscarriage can occur at any time during the pregnancy whether you have a test or not. Even one within two weeks of testing could be a 'natural miscarriage' as these also tend to occur earlier rather than later in the pregnancy.

# Processing of the Specimen

The chorionic tissue is placed into a dish or flask containing a special fluid. It is examined either with a low-power microscope or with the naked eye to see if there is adequate material. The aim is to obtain a minimum of 10 mg of villi from the placenta for processing. Where possible, it is preferable that this is taken immediately to the laboratory. A delay could reduce the success rate in growing the cells.

In the laboratory the chorionic villi are carefully dissected to remove any decidual cells, those from the mother which line the uterus and are often also aspirated during CVS. Either or both of the following methods are then used:

(i)   the chromosomes are looked at either without culturing or by culturing for a short period of up to 24 hours.

(ii)  the specimen is cultured for one week or more prior to processing. The cells are taken from the incubator (harvested) when adequate numbers of colonies of cells have grown.

When CVS first became available the first method was used which provided virtually immediate results. It was discovered, however, that occasionally the chromosome result was different from that of the baby. Many laboratories now use this method plus follow with the long-term method to confirm the results. Others use only one of the two methods. In the first method, the lining cells of the villi of the placenta (the cytotrophoblastic cells) are analysed while in the long-term method the core of the villi (the mesenchymal cells) are analysed. For complex reasons associated with the early development of these two tissues, the chromosomes can occasionally differ.

# Waiting for the Results

Laboratories that use the long-term culture will usually provide a final result within ten to twenty days. If the laboratory uses the direct preparation then this result would be available in less than one week. The time to process the results therefore varies with the technique used by the laboratory; but specimens also take differing lengths of times to grow. Laboratory work on the samples is time-consuming, one technician processing only about five a week. Overload on laboratory resources often delays the results. Generally, the result is available by 13 weeks pregnancy which is still up to seven weeks earlier than amniocentesis.

# Test Failure

If CVS is unsuccessful it is for one of two reasons — the operator failed to obtain an adequate specimen (technical failure) or the laboratory failed to produce an adequate result (laboratory failure). Both of these failure rates are higher with CVS than amniocentesis. Only about 1 per cent of women who have an amniocentesis will need a repeat test, whereas with CVS it is between 2 and 10 per cent, being closer to 2 per cent in expert hands.

CVS can be a more difficult technique than amniocentesis, hence the higher technical failure rate. With experience, the operator learns to circumvent the difficulties or anticipate difficulties which are likely to result in a failed test. Even so, experienced centres have a failure rate of between 1 per cent and 6 per cent for transcervical CVS and about 1.5 per cent for transabdominal CVS.

Difficulties are expected with a transcervical approach if there is a sharp bend in the cavity of the uterus or cervix. In early pregnancy the axis of a pregnant woman's uterus can be sharply bent forwards (anteverted) or backwards (retroverted). A fibroid (a thickening of the wall of the uterus) may cause a similar obstruction if it is low in the uterus, rendering the test difficult or impossible. The most difficult transabdominal CVS is the unusual situation when the uterus is tilted backwards (retroverted) and all of the placenta inserted into the back wall of the uterus. With experience, most of the difficulties discussed above may be circumvented. It has been suggested that all centres should have both techniques available because what is a difficult approach for one technique may be a fairly straightforward procedure for the alternate one.

Occasionally the laboratory receives a good specimen but none of the cells from the placenta grow. This happens in up to 2 per cent of specimens and prevents chromosome analysis. If the test does fail then the alternatives are to repeat the CVS, or have an amniocentesis. Whichever of the two methods is chosen, seldom does the second specimen fail to grow.

There are an additional two potential sources of error which can cause confusing results. Maternal cell contamination (the growth of cells from the mother instead of the baby) results in an analysis of the mother's chromosomes. Now that laboratories have become experienced at processing samples and meticulously removing any of the mother's tissues from the specimen, this is a rare occurrence. Another occasional problem is mosaicism. This is when different cells analysed in the laboratory have differing chromosomes, a condition occurring in a small percentage of people. The outcome for the baby depends on what the chromosome types are and the proportion of each type of cell. The CVS may occasionally show mosaicism even when this is not present in the baby. Experts often have a good idea whether the mosaicism is likely to be affecting the baby by looking at the pattern of the mixture of cells. Some mixtures of cells seen after CVS are so rare in liveborn babies that further testing usually shows that it is not present. Mosaicism occurs in approximately 1 per cent of CVS's and can readily be sorted out if an amniocentesis is performed.

Occasionally the test results are ambiguous or later prove to be incorrect. These may be 'false positives' when an abnormal result is obtained in a normal baby or 'false negatives' when a normal result is obtained in a baby with abnormal chromosomes. Most false positives are quickly detected by the laboratory as the abnormality is not seen in living pregnancies and follow-up amniocentesis is recommended. False negatives are very rare indeed.

Table 7.2 summarizes the chance of failure of CVS attributable to the causes outlined above. It shows that 2.2–10 per cent of women will require further testing either with a repeat CVS or amniocentesis. The chance that further testing is required depends mostly on the expertise of the doctor, as technical failures are potentially the largest group — it is at the lower end of the range in most experienced centres.

TABLE 7.2   REASONS FOR FAILURE OF CVS TESTING

| | |
|---|---|
| Inadequate or no specimen | 1–6% |
| Cells do not grow | 0.4–2% |
| Doubtful result | 0.8–2% |
| *Total* | 2.2–10% |

# CVS in Multiple Pregnancy

CVS can be performed in twin pregnancies but not usually if there are three or more babies. It is reasonable to perform CVS on twins if there are clearly two placentas both of which are accessible. In general, however, many believe twins to be a relative contraindication to the test.

# Questions

DOES CVS CAUSE THE BABY TO MOVE?   During CVS you may see the baby moving on the ultrasound screen but these are spontaneous — CVS has no influence on them. The needle is outside the pregnancy sac so the baby does not have any sensation or awareness of its presence.

IS CVS AS ACCURATE AS AMNIOCENTESIS?   If an abnormal result is produced with either test then it can be relied upon to be accurate. The doubtful CVS results are usually obvious to the laboratory and these can nearly always be cleared up by having an amniocentesis later.

## CAN CVS PICK UP AS MUCH AS AMNIOCENTESIS?
These two tests are as good as each other for diagnosing chromosomal abnormalities. Spina bifida cannot be diagnosed by CVS but most people having a CVS are at very low risk of having a baby with spina bifida. Spina bifida can also be diagnosed with ultrasound.

## DO MORE PEOPLE CHOOSE CVS OR AMNIOCENTESIS?
The most popular choice depends on local expertise. In centres with expertise in CVS it is found that more and more women are choosing this method.

## CAN MY CELLS GROW AT CVS INSTEAD OF THE BABY'S?
While this can happen, with modern techniques it very rarely does.

## CAN I HAVE CVS IF I HAVE BEEN BLEEDING?
A woman who has vaginal bleeding in early pregnancy has an increased chance of miscarriage even when the pregnancy appears healthy on ultrasound. Her 'background' risk is therefore higher than that of a woman who has had no bleeding. Whether performing a CVS in this situation also results in an increased risk of the test itself is uncertain. One reasonable policy is that if there has been no bleeding in the week prior to the proposed CVS and the pregnancy appears healthy on ultrasound then the test is unlikely to cause an increased risk of miscarriage.

## IF MISCARRIAGE OCCURS AFTER CVS WHEN WOULD IT HAPPEN?
Because miscarriages occur whether or not you have a CVS, there is no clear answer to this question. A miscarriage can occur at any time and there is no way of telling if the CVS caused it. Overall, there is a slight increase in miscarriage rate after either CVS or amniocentesis. It is usually recommended that you reduce your level of activity for the 12 to 24 hours following CVS but after this time there is little purpose in taking extra precautions.

## WHICH IS SAFEST — TRANSCERVICAL OR TRANSABDOMINAL CVS?
There is little difference in the risks of these two techniques. The risks depend more on who performs the procedure and their level of experience and skill. The doctor who is to carry out your test could tell you his or her results.

# 8 MAKING THE DECISIONS

Prenatal testing has become one of the more controversial areas in medicine. Along with in vitro fertilization, it has become a symbol to many of science's zeal to gain control over the future evolution of the human species. Terms like 'designer baby' and 'perfect product' are regularly applied to the aims of testing. Newspapers carry stories about women who refuse tests because they believe parents should accept children the way they are. Testing is criticized because it turns the birth experience into yet another consumer activity, or because it interferes with maternal attachment to the developing baby.

It is in this kind of environment, often sensationalized and confusing, that women are called upon to make some tough decisions. Should they let nature take its course and accept whatever child is delivered? Or should they put their already-loved and nurtured babies at additional risk to exclude some abnormalities? This chapter aims to help you go through the decision-making process and relates the experiences of some couples who have already considered their options. Our major concern is the level of informed consent given to the procedures. Whether you decide to have a test and which one, whether you decide to terminate the pregnancy on an abnormal result, depends on your circumstances. The decisions to be made are yours; there are no hard and fast rules.

Prenatal testing undoubtedly gives women the chance to exclude some of the uncertainties and anxieties surrounding pregnancy. But it does raise other uncertainties and issues which should be discussed within society. Now that the technology is widely available and relatively safe, should every couple have the right to testing?

What role should a doctor play in giving advice in such a medically and ethically complex area? How should parents act when uncertainties are raised by chromosome analysis and when it is difficult to predict what a child will be like from some results? This chapter also looks briefly at some of the ethical concerns of those working in the area of prenatal diagnosis. Bio-ethics is a complex area attracting a wide range of opinion, and it is beyond the scope of this book to analyse it in detail. For those interested, a list of further reading is included at the end of this book.

# ▌Eligibility for testing

By far the largest group of women having babies are those under 35 with no previous histories of genetic abnormalities. For these women, the risk of having a baby with a chromosome abnormality is so low that most doctors consider the additional risk of miscarriage of 0.5 to 1.0 per cent carried by genetic testing to be unwarranted. Unless there are other indications such as an affected baby having previously been delivered, a history of repeated miscarriages or structural abnormalities seen at ultrasound, most women of this age are limited to a scan. There are some, however, who are so anxious about the risk of abnormalities that they ask for testing at a younger age. The reasoning of one woman, Penny, who at 33 had an amniocentesis for her first child, shows the difficulty of imposing strict age limits.

> I had done a lot of work with retarded children and a number of their parents were quite young. Just because I was a couple of years younger than the usual testing time I didn't think that was sufficient guarantee that my baby would be all right. I knew my life options would mean continuing working and a disabled child would make this difficult. I had thought through the issue, and I decided I was prepared to terminate the pregnancy if it was a Down syndrome baby.

The results were normal but unfortunately Penny's baby was still-born. Pregnant again a year later, she again pushed for testing despite the trauma of already having lost a baby.

I knew it would be awful, but just because I had lost one baby didn't mean I wanted a retarded child. There was a lot of opposition from women in my support group who had also lost babies. Some were so desperate to have another child, they said: 'Give me one no matter what is wrong with it. I still wasn't considered to be in the high risk group and it was much harder to get a test than 12 months before. My obstetrician was supportive but he had to sales talk the pathologist and operator.

Situations such as Penny's have raised one of the major issues amongst service providers: should there be a strict age cut-off point or should informed parents be autonomous in their decision? Because of the labour-intensive nature and expense of the laboratory processing, many centres have imposed fairly strict limits on who can be tested. Recently, however, there has been a tendency for greater leeway, particularly with privately insured patients.

On the surface, it would seem equitable to give all informed parents the right to such procedures. But there are several strong arguments against making testing more readily available. Most women want to have everything they perceive will help ensure a healthy pregnancy. In one study, the risks of amniocentesis were explained to a group of low-risk women under 35, yet 85 per cent wanted to have the test. If offered such a test when in an emotionally vulnerable state during pregnancy, it may be difficult for a woman to make an informed decision based on the relative risks. Another argument is based on the cost of a test, which in most Western countries is equivalent to about an average week's wage. If the public foots the bill, governments expect to see a cost benefit to the testing and this is difficult to demonstrate in low-risk groups.

The other major issue affecting eligibility for testing, is the attitude of parents towards abortion. Many centres argue that it is unnecesssarily risky to carry out testing, unless you are prepared to terminate your pregnancy on an unfavourable result. Others, however, say there are strong arguments in favour of testing high-risk couples even when the detection of an abnormality would not lead to pregnancy termination. If the baby is diagnosed as abnormal, the news may be better taken in the doctor's office than at the stressful time of birth. Also, parents who choose to raise such a child will gain time for preparation. For Wendy, who found she was carrying a Down syndrome child, it gave her the chance to reset her goals.

> I was advised that it was medically unsound to have a test unless you were prepared to act on the result. This was because of the risk of miscarriage. So my decision to have an amniocentesis was not made lightly. When I eventually decided against termination, I found the testing had been very valuable. Through that knowledge I had the chance to reset my goals before Sarah was born. In my decision-making, I had the normal dream of a child who would go to university and have a successful, happy life. Many parents' hopes are dashed anyway on those dreams. Instead of that, I had the time to develop positive alternatives to build on.

# ▌Should I have a Test?

Table 8.1 outlines the major factors you should consider in deciding if a test is right for you. Advanced age is by far the most significant one, accounting for up to 90 per cent of women who are tested. At the age of 36 the probability of detecting a Down syndrome baby is about one in 200, the same as the risk of miscarriage attributed to amniocentesis. If you are above this age, you will be eligible for testing. If you are 36 or less but still wish to be tested you should discuss your concerns with your obstetrician. In some areas, blood tests are available for young pregnant women which will indicate if you are at increased risk of carrying a baby with a chromosome abnormality. If so, you will be offered an amniocentesis (see chapter 9).

Other influences that will affect your decision are your attitudes towards the risks of the tests, abortion and bringing up a child with abnormalities. If there is a history of genetic disorder in your family, this will have a major impact on your decision-making.

## ▌ASSESSMENT OF RISKS

Comparing statistical risks is fraught with problems. While it is convenient to say that at about age 36 the risk of miscarriage from

TABLE 8.1   FACTORS TO CONSIDER BEFORE DECIDING WHETHER TO
HAVE A TEST

| | **Amniocentesis / CVS** | **No test** |
|---|---|---|
| Age <35* | Performed if parents especially concerned | Favoured by balance of risks |
| Age 35–36 | Balance of risks depends on how the figures are assessed | |
| Age ≥37 | Favoured by balance of risks | If refused for reasons below |
| Parents' attitude | Wish to lower the chance of raising a child with an abnormality, so would accept abortion<br>*or*<br>Wishes time to accept an abnormality if present | Would accept a baby no matter what<br>*or*<br>Absolute moral, religious or other objection to abortion<br>*or*<br>Objection to pre-natal testing because it focuses on the disability not the baby's individuality |
| Risk of miscarriage | Accepts the low risk of test | Accepts no increased risk |

* The age is usually taken as the age you will be at the time the baby is due to deliver.

amniocentesis is equal to that of detecting a Down syndrome baby, in many ways this is a false comparison. Are the outcomes equal? On the one hand, you have the loss of a baby and on the other a lifetime spent looking after a disabled person. Studies have shown that many women are prepared to accept an even higher risk of miscarriage to guard against bringing an abnormal baby into the world. For others, especially those who have spent years trying to conceive, have had repeated miscarriages or suffered the death of a baby, any additional risk may seem too high. If you belong to this group, you might consider relying on ultrasound which in the best hands can detect many of those babies with major abnormalities without putting your pregnancy at risk.

# ■ ATTITUDES TOWARDS ABORTION

This book stresses that testing is a decision to be made by parents, not the doctor. It should be made after full counselling that covers individually the risks, limitations and emotional stress involved. For at the crux of prenatal testing is the couple's attitude towards abortion. Chromosomal abnormalities, if found, cannot be cured, the only choice is whether or not to have an abortion. It may help you to know about society's attitudes towards abortion. While it is still a contentious issue, a majority favour a couple's right to abortion.

A study by the Australian National University showed that 86 per cent of Australians approved of abortion if the baby might be defective; 76 per cent of Catholics approved. In the USA, 76 per cent approve of abortion for this reason, compared with 86 per cent in Great Britain.

It will help you to discuss beforehand what course you would take in the case of an abnormal result. As mentioned earlier, even if you are opposed to abortion, testing can be helpful. The odds favour a normal outcome which will help still some of your fears; if the result is abnormal, it will give you a valuable few months for preparation.

# ■ HISTORY OF GENETIC DISORDERS

For those couples with a previously affected child or a history of genetic disorder in their family, the decision to have testing is generally taken much more easily. In fact, many such couples would remain childless, if it were not for the availability of prenatal diagnosis. For couples who have previously given birth to a baby with

Down syndrome, the chance of a second baby with a chromosome abnormality rises to 1 per cent if the mother is under 35. Above this age, the risk is double the normal one associated with the specific age. When she became pregnant at 30, Heather did not fall into any of the high-risk groups for testing. She gave birth to a baby with Trisomy 18 who died 23 hours later. Again pregnant at 33, she was immediately offered an amniocentesis.

> I definitely wanted one. My chances of having another baby with a chromosome abnormality had increased from one in 1000 to one in 100. I was quite prepared to accept a miscarriage rate of one in 200 to avoid a recurrence. I think amniocentesis is a valuable test. I would have spent the whole pregnancy being worried if it were not for the reassurance of the test.

The risk of recurrence of other abnormalities is even higher: for spina bifida, it is 3 per cent after the first affected baby. One woman, whose first two babies were found to have spina bifida, terminated both pregnancies. After three years she became pregnant again, this time with a risk of 10 per cent of recurrence. Without amniocentesis, she would not have chanced the third pregnancy. Luckily, the results were normal as was her child. Those with a family history of a gene disorder can be at even greater risk. Maria and Sergio, both carriers of the thalassaemia gene defect, had a chance of one in four of having a child with thalassaemia major like Maria's cousin.

> My cousin has been through hell. He's very sickly and has to have repeated blood transfusions. They don't give him much chance of living beyond thirty-two. I wouldn't want to put a child through that. If we didn't have the option of testing, we would not have had a family. I had decided to terminate the pregnancy if the baby was shown to be abnormal. We were very lucky, and never had to exercise this option. It gave us great peace of mind and allowed us to go ahead and have three healthy children.

# ▋ THE LIMITS OF TESTING

One important issue that has been reiterated throughout this book is that the decision to have testing and act upon the result only **lowers your chances** of having an abnormal baby. A normal test result does not guarantee a normal, healthy delivery. Some major abnormalities cannot be detected by any prenatal tests including ultrasound, and there may be complications later in pregnancy or during the birth that cannot be predicted. Many women lose sight of this in the euphoria of normal results. When Maria's first pregnancy was tested for thalassaemia, the results were normal.

> I had a fetal blood test when I was first pregnant at 24. It was terrible waiting the six days for the results. But we were ecstatic. She was fine, everything was fine. Then I lost her when she was stillborn at seven months for some reason unrelated to the test. It was a terrible shock.

# ▌ COMMON REASONS FOR REFUSING TESTING

The most common reason for refusing amniocentesis or CVS is because the couple is against abortion. Other reasons are the risks involved or because the woman feels safe, has a commitment to this particular child or believes she should take parenthood the way it comes.

# ▌ Should I have an Amniocentesis or CVS?

In deciding which technique to have, there are advantages on either side which should be weighed up. Table 8.2 outlines the differences between the two methods. The major advantage of amniocentesis is that it is still a safer method than CVS of testing your baby. It is for this reason that people who have spent a long time trying to have a baby often choose amniocentesis. The method also has a lower technical failure rate and is less prone to producing ambiguous results, so fewer women who have amniocentesis will require repeat testing. The only time amniocentesis is always used is in the uncommon situation when there is a higher than usual risk of a specific abnormality which cannot be diagnosed on CVS. Spina bifida is such an abnormality.

The disadvantage of amniocentesis is that it is performed rela-

TABLE 8.2    FACTORS TO CONSIDER IN CHOOSING CVS OR
AMNIOCENTESIS

|  | **CVS** | **Amniocentesis** |
|---|---|---|
| Risk of miscarriage from test | Approximately 1% | Approximately 0.5% |
| Usual time to have test | 9–11 weeks | 15–17 weeks |
| When results received | 11–14 weeks (before mother looks pregnant or feels movements) | 18–20 weeks (after mother has felt movements) |
| Discomfort | Usually mild | Minimal |
| Type of abortion if sought | Vaginal (curette only) | Bring on labour (prostaglandins) |
| Test failure (see Table 7.2) | 2.2–10% | Approx. 1% |
| Previous baby with spina bifida | No | Yes |
| Obstetric factors previous Caesarean sections | Preferred | Late diagnosis a disadvantage |
| weak cervix needing a suture | Result back before suture | Result back after suture |
| Major advantage | Avoids late abortion | Lowest risk |

tively late in pregnancy, and it is not until 18 to 20 weeks that the
diagnosis is obtained. By this stage you look pregnant and you are
very aware of your baby's movements. If the baby is abnormal and
you choose to have the pregnancy aborted it is therefore emotionally much tougher. It is also medically more difficult to abort a

pregnancy of 20 weeks than it is at the early stages. There are drugs which can reliably bring you into labour at this late stage, but this usually takes up to twenty-four hours and involves going through labour. As you would know that your baby is abnormal and could not survive, this is a very unpleasant experience. Many women when counselled about having an amniocentesis are not told what a termination will involve.

> I had decided to terminate the pregnancy if it was a Down syndrome baby. But I was never told what it means to have an abortion at this stage. When I discovered it would involve a delivery, this was very traumatic for me as I had already lost one baby at birth.
>
> I had already had one baby die soon after birth because of an extra chromosome. When the results came back from amniocentesis, my decision would be to terminate the pregnancy if necessary. But I don't think I appreciated what this meant. At 20 weeks, you have an almost viable baby. It got to the point, that if it had had the same chromosome abnormality I decided I would go through the pregnancy and let it die at birth.

Because the results of CVS are available so much earlier, this has become a popular test. Certainly anybody who has been unfortunate enough to have an abortion at 20 weeks because of an abnormality tends to choose a CVS subsequently.

> Our pregnancy was settled, and I was fit and healthy. It never occurred to us that anything could be wrong. We decided to have an amniocentesis, anyway. When the obstetrician rang, we thought it was to change the appointment. We couldn't believe Ben had a sex chromosome abnormality. The obstetrician had said termination would be difficult, but I didn't realize just how terrible it would be or that it would involve twenty hours of labour. It was particularly awful because of the drugs and the way it was induced. If I had known, I would have chosen a CVS.

Those who have undergone CVS have a marked reduction in the level of anxiety and depression from the time they obtain their results. This occurs even though they are still at risk of miscarriage. From this time they are able to become attached to their babies. By contrast, those who have amniocentesis remain anxious until they receive their results at 20 weeks. Feelings of attachment are suppressed for half the pregnancy, the following comment being typical of many who undergo the procedure:

> I hid my pregnancy until the amnio results came back. I have contact with hundreds of people through my job and none of them commented on my pregnancy until I announced it at 20 weeks.

# Should I find out the Sex?

A chromosome analysis also indicates the sex of the baby and this is written on the laboratory report. Your doctor can tell you the sex if you wish. There is a range of attitudes on this subject. Some say that knowing the sex will take some of the excitement out of the birth and begin the process of sex stereotyping even earlier. Others believe in having all the information available on their baby.

# Should I have an Abortion?

The decision to have an abortion ultimately lies with the couple involved. If you are unfortunate enough to get an abnormal result on the genetic tests, you will want to know how seriously this will affect your child. Unfortunately, chromosome analysis will not always give a clear picture of the severity of the disabilities afflicting your child. Ultrasound will assist in assessing structural abnormality but will tell you nothing about mental development or organ function. Expert advice from geneticists or pediatric specialists will fill in some of the gaps, while self-help groups will willingly share with you the experiences of parents who have decided to bring up children with abnormalities.

If the abnormality is one of the trisomies such as Down syndrome or a serious congenital defect like spina bifida, almost everyone decides to have an abortion. Most couples if given a choice cannot bear the idea of bringing severely intellectually or physically disabled children into the world. Even these abnormalities, where there is known to be a marked reduction in the quality of life, cause some parents much heartbreak in coming to a decision. One woman, who eventually decided to terminate her pregnancy on a Down syndrome result, said:

> There are enormous ethical issues at stake, if we are to say people shouldn't live because they don't meet expectations. But these are abstract ideas. I couldn't stand to watch a child of mine being treated as the intellectually disabled are in our society.

There are very few women, like Wendy mentioned earlier, who make a decision to continue their pregnancies. Her experiences and the kind of research she undertook, may help you in your decision-making. At 42, Wendy discovered through amniocentesis that her first baby had Down syndrome.

> The results came back faster than expected, in less than three weeks. I went though a process of gathering information so that my decision would be an informed one. I visited schools and centres for those with Down syndrome. I went out with social workers. Personally I couldn't see any difference between a living person at five months and one at nine months and I wasn't going to take a life without knowing the extent of the disabilities. The situation was closely monitored with ultrasound to see if there were any major heart abnormalities. It seemed that it was 90 per cent sure that the heart was normal. It took me ten days to decide. Knowing that she would have a reasonable quality of life, I believed I didn't have the right to take it. Just because she didn't reach the norm, should she be culled? Her father left me as soon as I made the decision. He couldn't cope and I didn't see him again until Sarah was born. I had prepared myself that she would be healthy and it was an excellent birth. Knowing she was a Down syndrome baby did not detract from the experience. My goals by then were different and I had reset all my aspirations for her. Her father came to the birth and once he saw her, I couldn't get her out of his arms. She's now six months old, a delightful little girl that her father sees once a week. I'm very happy about my decision.

There are other conditions such as sex chromosome abnormalities where the range of disability is wider still. Some children may show few abnormalities, others are mentally delayed. This uncertainty presents couples with a difficult decision; about half deciding to terminate while the rest proceeding with the pregnancy. If a couple desperately want a child and have had trouble conceiving, they may find the risk of lower intelligence and infertility bearable. If, on the other hand, this is an accidental pregnancy and the couple have several other healthy children, they may decide to terminate the pregnancy. If they have strong academic interests, the couple might not be able to cope with the idea of a child incapable of gaining a university education.

In general, the law is interpreted as allowing an abortion if there is a specific risk to the mental or physical well-being of the mother. In practice, it is usually liberally interpreted. This places doctors, most of whom believe in the autonomy of parents to make their own decisions, in a difficult situation. It can be very hard to convince anxious parents that many minor conditions such as a cleft palate and lip are treatable. Some people wish to abort on this diagnosis.

As the technology increases in sophistication, so will the danger that parents will want to terminate pregnancies for even more minor abnormalities. Much of the opposition to prenatal testing rests on this point; on the attempt to create perfect babies. Where should the line be drawn? There could be dire consequences for future society if sex selection were used as a common basis for abortion. In some Asian countries such as China this has occurred, leading to a legal ban on the practice. Although it occurs rarely in Western countries, some doctors have become so concerned that they do not reveal the baby's sex to parents.

If you decide to have an abortion, it is likely to be a traumatic experience, particularly when it is a much wanted baby. Whether at 12 or 20 weeks, abortion still involves the loss of a baby. Many women find that the community does not appreciate the bonding they have with that particular child, and receive comments like 'Don't worry, you'll have another one.' You will need time to say goodbye to the baby and to rally support. Some women ask for the diagnosis to be confirmed after the abortion. They are concerned that the doctor has made a mistake and that all this technology is not really looking after them. Frequently, a biopsy can be carried out on the baby which gives some women reassurance that they have made the right decision. As with the loss of any baby, you are likely to go through a grieving process and have increased anxiety with future pregnancies.

# ▌The Role of the Doctor

Two of the major dilemmas for doctors working in prenatal diagnosis are striking a balance between full disclosure of information and causing inappropriate parental anxiety and the issue of non-directive counselling. Everybody agrees in principle with the full disclosure of results to parents. But there are borderline situations such as a mosaic result at CVS in which there are only one or two abnormal cells as against 150 normal ones, which are extremely unlikely to have any impact on the baby. Yet when a doctor tries to explain this, parents commonly have such an extreme fear of abnormality that the slightest suggestion of a problem confirms their worst fears. There may be no medical uncertainty about a result, but conveying this to parents can be difficult.

A case that illustrates the point well is the distress of Margaret, whose baby was found at amniocentesis to have a pericentric inversion of chromosome 9. She was assured that this inversion had never been known to produce any abnormalities in babies and was considered a normal variant. Family members were tested for the inversion, and the variant was found in both her husband and his mother. This did not reassure Margaret — in fact, she kept looking for defects in their personalities and physical attributes which might be associated with the inversion. At one stage, she thought it might be connected with the fact that both were a little hard of hearing. She worried for her entire pregnancy, until the baby was born and seen to be fine.

The majority of doctors involved in the area of prenatal diagnosis strongly advocate non-directive counselling; that results, risks and options should be presented as objectively as possible. Even with the best will in the world, it is often difficult for a counsellor to avoid indicating his or her views. Many of the concepts are complex and couples tend to seek direction from experts in the field.

# 9 WHY NOT JUST TEST THE MOTHER'S BLOOD?

We would all like to see medicine develop to the point where a simple blood test on the mother would enable any abnormality in the baby to be detected. While genetic analysis is advancing rapidly, this aim is still beyond the dreams of even the greatest optimist. However, blood tests which indicate that further testing of the baby should be carried out are available. In this chapter we will look at what is available now and what may be available in the future.

Amniocentesis and CVS have developed to the point that they are both widely available and safe techniques for accurate diagnosis of chromosomal abnormalities. If you are at high risk of having a baby with a chromosomal abnormality, these techniques are available to you. If, however, like 90 per cent of the population, your chance of having a such a baby is very small, then these tests are unlikely to be· available to you.

The irony of this situation is that most Down syndrome babies are not detected prior to birth. This is because women usually have their children before the age of 35 when the individual risks of having such a baby are considered too low to warrant testing. Together, however, these younger 'low-risk' mothers give birth to 65 per cent of Down syndrome babies. We are learning to detect some of the subtle differences between normal and Down syndrome babies at an 18 week ultrasound scan, but these criteria are only just now being developed. The differences are difficult to detect and it will be some time before we know the proportion of Down syndrome babies who can be detected with ultrasound alone. If we are to improve the detection rate then all pregnant women should have some other 'screening test'.

A screening test that involved something simple like testing the mother's blood would be ideal; especially if it were cheap enough so that all pregnant women could have it performed. It might not be perfect. It might miss some Down syndrome babies and give some 'false positive' results, i.e. an abnormal result when the mother is carrying a normal baby. But women with an 'abnormal' blood test could then be offered amniocentesis or CVS to confirm the diagnosis. The aim would be to improve the detection rate for babies with chromosomal abnormalities.

Two sorts of blood tests have been suggested as screening methods for Down syndrome. The first involves looking for cells from the placenta which escape into the mother's circulation, and the second is based on proteins and hormones which cross from the baby into the mother's circulation.

# ▌Baby's Cells in the Mother's Circulation

Throughout pregnancy there are occasions when cells from the baby's placenta and bloodstream enter the mother's circulation. These placental cells (the medical name is trophoblast cells) pass into the mother's veins around the uterus and travel up towards the heart. They are then pumped with the blood through the lungs and the rest of the body. Samples taken from the veins of mothers' arms have contained trophoblast cells. The two major questions to be answered are: can a chromosome analysis of the baby be obtained from these cells, and how often during pregnancy can these cells be detected?

Unfortunately, despite some early optimistic reports, there are some problems with this test which must be overcome. Any cells entering the mother's circulation are filtered twice before they get to her arm. They must pass through the liver on the way to the heart, and then through the lungs before being again pumped around the body. Both the liver and the lungs tend to remove cells such as trophoblast from the circulation. There are likely, therefore, to be far fewer cells present in the arm than there were originally entering the circulation. Although sophisticated new techniques can sometimes detect the sex of the baby, attempts to analyse baby's chromosomes from these cells have so far been unsuccessful. For the time being, therefore, we need to look elsewhere for our screening test. A new method, whereby antibody-coated metal beads attach to any cells from the baby then a magnet is used to isolate them, shows promise for the future.

# ▌Hormone and Biochemical Tests

The combined use of hormone and biochemical tests on the mother's blood is a very promising method of detecting Down syndrome and spina bifida. The tests described below are already being used in some centres and in the next few years are likely to gain wide acceptance in clinical practice.

## ▌ALPHA-FETOPROTEIN (AFP) TEST

Alpha-fetoprotein (AFP) is a protein made by your baby that circulates in its bloodstream to help maintain fluid balance. Tiny amounts also enter your own circulation during pregnancy, the levels rising as your pregnancy advances.

For many years the level of AFP in the amniotic fluid has been used as a test for spina bifida. In spina bifida there is an opening in the baby's skin between the spinal canal and the amniotic fluid. The level of AFP is very much higher in the fluid around the spinal cord (the cerebrospinal fluid), so a spina bifida causes more to pass into the amniotic fluid. This results in much higher levels also finding their way into the mother's circulation.

Many Western countries routinely offer tests of maternal serum AFP (i.e. the level of alpha-fetoprotein in the mother's blood stream) at 15 to 18 weeks. This allows the detection of 95 per cent of babies with anencephaly and 70 per cent with spina bifida.

Most babies whose mothers have a high serum AFP do *not* have spina bifida. It is a screening test which does not aim to be totally accurate but merely selects a group of babies who require further testing. Occasionally other conditions such as twins or a deficiency in the baby's abdominal wall (an exomphalos) may cause a raised serum AFP. It may also indicate a pregnancy which is further advanced than expected.

If the maternal serum AFP is high, further tests are carried out, the first being an ultrasound examination. This will detect many of the causes such as spina bifida, twins, or an exomphalos. If the ultrasound gives a normal result and the baby's size is appropriate for dates, then amniocentesis may be suggested to test the AFP in the amniotic fluid, as this is a more precise test. Usually, however, ultrasound will identify any defect.

Babies with Down syndrome tend to produce a slightly lower maternal serum AFP at 15 to 18 weeks than normal babies. There is, however, a substantial overlap in the AFP levels between normal babies and those with Down syndrome. Just as the majority of those mothers with a high AFP levels do not have a spina bifida baby, so the majority of those with low AFP levels do not have a Down syndrome baby. Their chances are raised, however. If maternal serum AFP is found to be low, an ultrasound examination is first performed to confirm the dates, then an amniocentesis offered to test the baby for Down syndrome. In some places, pregnant women are offered amniocentesis based on the risk of Down syndrome calculated using maternal serum AFP combined with the woman's age.

Although it does increase the detection rate, routine measurement of maternal serum AFP in this way still does not pick up most babies with Down syndrome. Research workers have therefore continued to seek more efficient ways of detection. Note that while maternal serum AFP can be measured in a laboratory no matter where you live, unless there is a local screening programme in place for all pregnant women it is probably not worth being tested. Unless the laboratory carries out large numbers of tests, it is difficult for it to define its normal ranges clearly enough to be useful for testing for spina bifida and Down syndrome.

# ▌ COMBINED TESTING ON SERUM AFP AND HORMONES

It has been shown that by using a combination of blood tests on pregnant women, all taken at 16 to 18 weeks, one can improve the detection rate for Down syndrome. It is known that mothers carrying a Down syndrome baby tend to have different levels of two other substances in their blood. These are human chorionic gonadotrophin (HCG) — the hormone that is being measured in a pregnancy test — and an oestrogen called 'unconjugated oestriol'. This hormone is sometimes tested for at the end of pregnancy to check the baby's growth. It has been shown that these four, the mother's age, high levels of HCG, and low levels of AFP and unconjugated oestriol, can be combined to provide the most efficient way of screening for Down syndrome yet devised. If the 5 per cent of pregnant women with the most abnormal combination have an amniocentesis, then 60 per cent of Down syndrome babies will be detected. While not infallible, this combination is a big improvement on current methods. If all women over 35 have an amniocentesis or CVS, only 35 per cent of Down syndrome babies will be detected because most are born to younger mothers and these are missed. Using the combined method, about 2 per cent of those going on to have an amniocentesis will have a Down syndrome baby detected. Thus, most pregnant women with abnormal results from blood screening tests carry a normal baby, but the chance that it has Down syndrome is increased.

Doubtless a great deal more work will be done in this area. Different combinations of tests will be devised which will increase the pick-up rate for Down syndrome. As we discussed in Chapter 4, ultrasound can be used to detect a proportion of the Down syndrome babies and it is likely that eventually some ultrasound findings will be included in the formula to calculate which women should be offered an amniocentesis.

There are several difficulties with commencing screening of all pregnant women for Down syndrome as proposed. Those women who are already eligible to have CVS or amniocentesis, such as those above the current age limit of 35 to 37, are likely to continue to wish to have these more reliable tests. It is possible that all women over a certain age, such as 38, might still be offered CVS or amniocentesis even if their hormone and protein levels are normal.

A major problem with such a screening programme is a technical one. The organization involved in explaining the test to women, establishing a good collection and laboratory service, then feeding back the results is a mammoth project. Nevertheless, this is the most efficient system to detect Down syndrome and such programmes are being established.

Another difficulty with such a screening programme is that the tests are not taken until 16 weeks pregnancy. If taken earlier, the tests do not allow discrimination between normal babies and those with spina bifida or Down syndrome. By the time the results of blood tests and amniocentesis are available, the pregnancy is likely to be at least 20 weeks. Medically, an abortion can still be performed at this stage if this is the parent's request but in some places it may be beyond the legal time limit and as discussed in Chapter 8 is often traumatic. The enormous advantage of CVS in providing early diagnosis of abnormalities is lost by this method of screening. It is possible that in time tests may be found which can be carried out very early in pregnancy.

# ▌Questions

SURELY THERE MUST BE SOMETHING WRONG WITH MY BABY IF MY SERUM AFP IS ABNORMAL?    It is not really correct to look on your test as abnormal but merely in the high or low range which means that there is a higher risk of an abnormality being present. More than 95 per cent of the people that have a test outside the normal range have an absolutely healthy baby.

IF MY BABY HAS AN ABNORMALITY CAUSING THE HIGH OR LOW SERUM AFP, WILL YOU BE ABLE TO FIND IT?    If the test shows a low AFP level and has been caused by your baby having Down syndrome then the amniocentesis will show this. If the AFP level is high then ultrasound can be expected to pick up around 95 per cent of the babies with spina bifida. If the ultrasound is normal, then some doctors would then also suggest that you have amniocentesis which occasionally detects a spina bifida missed on the scan. With follow-up testing using ultrasound and possibly amniocentesis, it is most unlikely that a baby with spina bifida would be missed.

# 10 OTHER TESTS OCCASIONALLY USED

In this book we have concentrated on ultrasound, CVS and amniocentesis as these are the most widely used tests to look for abnormalities or genetic disease. The aim of this chapter is to complete the picture by examining other methods of visualizing your baby, and other invasive tests currently used or likely to be used in the near future. We will conclude with a short segment on treatment of babies with abnormalities before birth.

## Other Ways of looking at your Baby

### X-RAYS

X-rays are still occasionally used in pregnancy, although ultrasound has usurped many of its roles. In the non-medical community there remains a widespread concern that X-rays during pregnancy may cause abnormalities or cancer later in childhood. While at high doses both of these can happen, using modern X-ray equipment the dose of irradiation is very low. It is now believed that X-rays used for diagnosis will not cause these problems.

X-rays are used for three purposes in pregnancy:

(i)  To look at the baby for structural abnormalities, to see which way it is lying or to diagnose multiple pregnancy. Ultrasound has now virtually totally replaced the use of X-rays in these areas.

(ii)  To examine the size of the pregnant women's pelvis. Occasionally it is important to know the size of the pelvis before labour if, for example, the baby has a breech presentation (buttocks down), or if the mother has had a Caesarean section with an earlier baby. Ultrasound is not able to measure the pelvic size. When these X-rays are carried out, as much of the baby as possible is shielded from the X-rays so that it receives the minimum dose.

(iii) To investigate other diseases in pregnancy. If the pregnant woman has an illness in pregnancy, such as kidney disease, this may require investigation with X-rays. Wherever possible, the baby is shielded when the X-rays are taken.

The general principle is that X-rays are only used if their potential benefit is likely to far outweigh any risks.

## ■ MAGNETIC RESONANCE IMAGING (MRI)

This is a new and exciting tool for medicine which is likely to be used more and more. It has the advantage of showing tissue function whereas ultrasound cannot. The patient is placed in a large magnet, the magnet turned on and the energy released by the body's molecules measured when it is turned off. This very expensive equipment provides beautiful high-resolution images and is increasingly used for diagnosis of diseases. Its use in obstetrics has been limited because of the cost and because the still images produced are less versatile and useful than ultrasound. As it does not involve irradiation, it is believed to be safe. More work has to be done in this area before the technique can be used widely on the unborn baby.

# ■ Other Tests on Amniotic Fluid

## ■ FOR INFECTION

While most infections during pregnancy are known to be unlikely to damage the baby, there are several that may. German measles (rubella) was the first infection demonstrated to produce abnormalities in the baby and this still occurs occasionally in pregnancy. Other potentially damaging infections are cytomegalovirus (CMV) and toxoplasmosis, both more common but less hazardous than rubella. Rubella causes a rash and CMV and toxoplasmosis a prolonged flulike illness. If a pregnant woman has an illness suggestive of one of these, or contacts somebody with the disease, she can have a blood test. If the blood test is positive then amniocentesis or fetal blood sampling may be suggested to see if the baby developed the infection. Amniocentesis may also be used to look for infection if the membranes rupture early. If this occurs, infection is able to spread up into the uterus from the vagina.

# ▌ FOR BLOOD GROUP INCOMPATIBILITY

If there is a blood group incompatibility between the mother and baby (the commonest and best known one being Rhesus or Rh incompatibility), then routine tests on the mother's blood will detect it. Amniocentesis or fetal blood sample is often used to assess the severity of anaemia in the baby resulting from the blood group incompatibility. While these are performed late in pregnancy, the techniques and most of the risks are similar to those discussed in Chapter 6 and in this chapter respectively.

# ▌ FOR LUNG MATURITY

Lung immaturity of very premature babies presents their most common barrier to survival. Normal babies and adults produce fluid called surfactant which lines the air spaces to the lungs and prevents their collapse. Babies do not produce surfactant until about 34 weeks or sometimes even later. When an infant is likely to deliver early, amniocentesis may be performed to test for the presence of this surfactant in the amniotic fluid as a means of indicating if the baby is likely to have severe lung disease after birth. If surfactant is not present then an injection of steroids (cortisone) into the mother will cross the placenta and help the baby to produce it.

# ▌ Fetal Blood Sampling (FBS)

Fetal blood sampling is an ultrasound-guided technique shown in figure 10.1 in which a needle is passed through the skin and uterus of the pregnant women and into a blood vessel of the baby, usually in its umbilical cord, to withdraw blood. When used for chromosome testing, its major advantage is that a result is available in less than one week. The test is often called percutaneous umbilical blood sampling (PUBS) or cordocentesis. The main reasons for having FBS are:

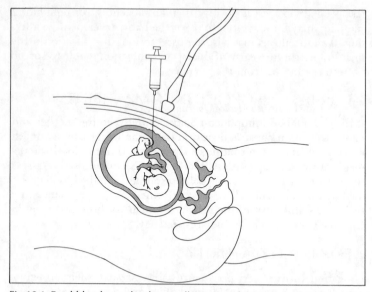

Fig 10.1 Fetal blood sample: the needle is passed into a vessel in the cord, usually at a point 1–2 cm from the placenta.

(i)    an at-risk pregnancy (e.g. age greater than 35) where the woman presents too late to allow laboratory processing of chromosomes in an amniocentesis specimen;
(ii)   an abnormality found on ultrasound that may be the result of an underlying chromosomal abnormality;
(iii)  a baby at high risk of a disease in to test for required for diagnosis — e.g. some cases of haemophilia and thalassaemia;
(iv)   some intra-uterine infections, e.g. toxoplasmosis;
(v)    a baby with markedly reduced growth, to test for an underlying chromosomal abnormality or for oxygen and carbon dioxide levels in the baby's blood;
(vi)   a major increase or decrease in amniotic fluid volume.

# ▌ TIMING OF FBS

Fetal blood sampling may be performed at any time after 16 weeks. In general it becomes easier later in pregnancy. There has been a report of its use as early as 12 weeks but the cord is very fine at this stage and generally it is not carried out until later.

# ■ WHO SHOULD PERFORM THE FETAL BLOOD SAMPLE?

A report in the *British Medical Journal* suggests that centres performing FBS should be doing at least 30 per year. Expertise is more easily maintained by a doctor whose practice includes amniocentesis and CVS. If you ask, the doctor should be able to give you an idea of the numbers performed and the miscarriage rate following the test in his/her practice.

# ■ THE PROCEDURE

A 20- to 22-gauge needle is passed under ultrasound guidance through the skin of the mother's abdomen, through the uterus and into the cord near the point where it connects with the placenta. The passage of the needle is either through the placenta and directly into the cord without entering the amniotic space, or into the amniotic space and then on into the cord. Once the needle is inside the cord it is manipulated until the tip enters one of the blood vessels and blood can be withdrawn into the syringe. Afterwards, the site in the cord that has been punctured is checked to ensure that bleeding is not occurring, and the baby's heartbeat is observed for any irregularity.

Blood may also be taken from a vessel within the baby's body instead of the umbilical cord, or directly from the baby's heart.

From the pregnant woman's point of view this procedure differs little from amniocentesis. No special preparation is required before the fetal blood sample. The procedure may take longer than amniocentesis as the operator must place the tip of the needle into a vessel in the cord. Following FBS there is no need to stay in hospital but you will be advised to go home and rest.

# ■ POSSIBLE COMPLICATIONS

The most important complication of the test is death of the baby due to the test. In experienced hands this occurs in approximately 1 to 2 per cent of cases. Other potential complications include persistent bleeding from the cord after withdrawal of the needle: bleeding usually stops within one minute. In rare cases there may be bleeding into the cord to produce a localized haematoma (blood collection). Following blood sampling the heart rate may slow but it usually returns to normal soon after. Other complications are potentially the same as for amniocentesis.

# ▌Biopsy of your Baby

The precision provided by ultrasound allows a piece of tissue from the baby to be removed with a needle. This is rarely done, but might be needed, for example, to do a skin biopsy of a baby who is at risk of a severe skin disease which would result in its death shortly after birth. The procedure of skin biopsy is similar to amniocentesis, with ultrasound providing the means to place the tip of the biopsy forceps against the skin where a small piece is taken. With appropriate equipment this is not usually difficult and therefore is not an unduly risky procedure for the baby, but because it is not commonly done, precise figures cannot be quoted. Usually there is little or no mark visible from where the skin was taken, after birth. Other parts may be biopsied, such as the liver, but this is rarely called for.

# ▌Fetoscopy

Ultrasound-guided procedures have virtually replaced fetoscopy, the passage of a telescope-like instrument through the abdomen and into the uterus to allow direct visualization of the baby, the cord and placenta. It has been used since 1973 for taking blood or other tissues, and for looking at some abnormalities which are difficult to diagnose using any other method. This procedure was technically difficult and took a great deal of experience, and the risk of miscarriage after the test was much higher than with ultrasound-guided procedures. Since the improved resolution of ultrasound equipment has allowed the detection of most abnormalities visualized by fetoscopy there is now little place for this technique.

# ▌Embryoscopy

Embryoscopy is the use of a telescope-like instrument which is passed into the vagina and through the cervix to provide direct visualization of the fetus. It is used in the first three months of pregnancy and provides spectacular moving pictures of the baby. It is currently used largely as a research tool in several specialized centres. There have been difficulties in developing good equipment. To see the baby the outside membrane around it must be ruptured, leaving only the inner sac which retains the fluid around the baby intact. There is concern that by rupturing the outside sac there may be unacceptable risk to the pregnancy, so it is not yet in widespread use. If the risks can be shown to be low it may well evolve into a useful technique.

# Intrauterine Treatment

Treatment of abnormalities before birth has aroused the curiosity and excitement of doctors and scientists in this field for many years. The concept of detecting an abnormality and then treating it to allow the delivery of a healthy baby must be the goal of any test in pregnancy. In this short section all that we can do is to introduce the concepts of treatment and briefly describe conditions which may be treated. It must be appreciated that very few abnormalities can be treated before birth.

The first and most straightforward method of treatment before birth is to give the mother a drug which will cross the placenta to the baby. This method has been used for many years to help premature babies' lungs mature before birth; if steroids are given to the mother they cross the placenta and result in the baby producing a fluid which lines the air cavities of the lungs and stops them collapsing after birth. If a baby's heartbeat is irregular, then appropriate drugs may be given to the mother to help regulate it.

The most successful direct treatment of complications in a baby prior to birth is blood transfusion. This is most commonly used where there is incompatibility between the baby's and the mother's blood resulting in the baby's red blood cells being destroyed. The baby can become very anaemic, its tissues become swollen with fluid and it can ultimately die. Injection of blood into the baby will prevent this happening and usually allow the delivery of a healthy baby. The blood may be injected into the abdomen of the baby and be slowly absorbed into its circulation or it may be injected directly into one of the blood vessels, usually in the umbilical cord. While these procedures may be technically difficult, in expert hands they will result in a high percentage of babies who would have otherwise died being delivered normal and healthy.

Other methods of direct treatment of the baby prior to birth have been less successful. The two most commonly used have been on babies with hydrocephaly (water on the brain) and hydronephrosis (blocked outflow from the kidneys). In both situations there is a large collection of fluid which builds up in the affected area. Many such babies have been treated by placing a tube, called a shunt, with one end in the fluid collection and the other in the surrounding amniotic cavity. The drainage of such fluid collections may be technically successful, but often there has been such severe damage to the underlying organs that the baby has little or no chance of healthy survival after birth. Disappointing results have caused the virtual abandonment of treatment of hydrocephaly. A small group of those babies with blocked kidneys who are otherwise normal benefit from a drainage procedure.

The final method of treatment we will discuss is a surgical operation on an unborn baby. This requires making an incision into the abdomen of the mother, opening the uterus and partially removing the baby from the uterus. There are several centres in the world where this is being carried out for procedures such as inserting a shunt or repairing a hernia in the diaphragm of an unborn baby. There is still a large amount to be learnt both in selecting which babies would benefit from such an operation and in minimizing the risks to the mother, both in this and subsequent pregnancies. It is uncertain whether such operations will ever be in more widespread use.

# ▌Conclusion

**Of necessity, this book has dealt with the abnormal. Such problems are rare but they do occur. Many can be detected prenatally but no one should undergo the tests without knowing the risks and benefits involved. This book emphasizes the fact that you do have a choice and that it is only through knowledge that you will be able to exercise it.**

*There is no cure for birth and death save to enjoy the interval* (Santayana)

# FURTHER READING

B. Brambati, G. Simoni, S. Fabro (eds), *Chorionic villus sampling. Fetal diagnosis of genetic diseases in the first trimester*, Marcel Dekker Inc., New York, 1986.

A. Clegg, A. Woolett, *Twins: From conception to five years*, First Ballantine Books, New York 1988.

N. Clopton, *Caring for Your Child with Spina Bifida*, Eterna Press, Oak Brook, Ill., 1981.

M. A. England, *A Colour Atlas of Life Before Birth: Normal fetal development*, Wolfe Medical Publications, London, 1983.

J. Fletcher, D. Wertz, Ethical aspects of prenatal diagnosis: Views of U.S. Medical Geneticists, *Clinics in Perinatology*, 1987 14, 293–312.

R. J. M. Gardner and G. R. Sutherland, *Chromosome Abnormalities and Genetic Counselling*, Oxford Monographs in Medical Genetics No. 17, Oxford University Press, Oxford, 1989.

J. H. Lord, *No Time for Goodbyes; coping with sorrow, anger and injustice after a tragic death*, Pathfinder, Ventura, California, 1987.

R. Romero, G. Pilu, P. Jeanty, A. Ghidini, J. Hobbins *Prenatal Diagnosis of Congenital Abnormalities*, Appleton & Lange, Connecticut 1988.

B. K: Rothman, *The Tentative Pregnancy: Prenatal diagnosis and the future of motherhood*, Viking, New York, 1986.

M. J. Schleifer and S. D. Klein, *The Disabled Child and the Family: an exceptional parent reader*, The Exceptional Parent Press, Boston, 1985.

Simons, R. *After the Tears: parents talk about raising a child with a disability*, Harcourt Brace Jovanovich, San Diego, 1987.

# REFERENCES

Chapter 1

R. E. Scammon, and L. A. Calkins, *The Development and Growth of the External Dimensions of the Human Body in the Fetal Period*, University of Minnesota Press, Minneapolis; 1929.

B. K. Rothman, *The Tentative Pregnancy, Prenatal diagnosis and the future of motherhood* Viking, New York, 1986.

Chapter 2

D. Cox, B. Wittmann, M. Hess et al, 'The Psychological Impact of Diagnostic Ultrasound', *Obstet Gynecol* 1987, 70, 673–6.

A. Saari-Kemppainen, O. Karjalainen, P. Ylostalo, O. Heinonen, 'Ultrasound screening and perinatal mortality: Controlled trial of systematic one-stage screening in pregnancy, *Lancet* 1990, 386, 387–91.

S. B. Thacker, Quality of Controlled Clinical Trials. The case of imaging ultrasound in obstetrics; a review', *Br J Obstet Gynaecol 1985*, 92, 437–44.

Chapter 3

M. B. Braken, 'Ultrasonography in Antenatal Management: should it be a routine procedure?, *Fetal Ther* 1987, 20, 2–6.

D. Liebeskind, R. Bases, F. Mendez et al, 'Sister Chromatid Exchanges in Human Lymphocytes after Exposure to Diagnostic Ultrasound', *Science* 1979, 205, 1273–5.

C. R. Stark, M. Orleans, A. D. Haverkamp, and J. Murphy, 'Short- and long-term risks after exposure to diagnostic ultrasound in utero', *Obstet Gynecol* 1984, 63, 194–200.

L. Warsof and S. K. Sayegh, 'Ultrasound Diagnosis of Intrauterine Growth Retardation', *Fetal Therapy* 1987, 2, 31–6.

Chapter 4

E. Dreazen, F. Tessler, D. Sarti, B. F. Crandall, 'Spontaneous Resolution of fetal hydrocephalus', *J Ultrasound Med* 1989, 8, 155–7.

R. Romero, G. Pilu, P. Jeanty, A. Ghidini and J. Hobbins, *Prenatal Diagnosis of Congenital Anomalies*, Appleton & Lange, 1988.

H. Rosendahl, S. Kivinen, 'Antenatal Detection of Congenital Mal-formations by Routine Ultrasonography; *Obstet Gynecol* 1989, 73, 947–51

## Chapter 5

M. A. Ferguson-Smith, and J. R. W. Yates, 'Maternal Age-Specific Rates for Chromosome Aberrations and Factors Influencing Them: a report of a collaborative European study on 56,965 Amniocenteses, *Prenatal Diagnosis* 1984, 4, 5–44.

T. Fryers *The Epidemiology of Severe Intellectual Impairment*, Academic Press, London, 1984.

R. J. M. Gardner and G. R. Sutherland, *Chromosome Abnormalities and Genetic Counselling*, Oxford Monographs in Medical Genetics No. 17, Oxford University Press, Oxford, 1989.

B. E. Hashimoti, B. S. Mahony, R. A. Filly, et al, 'Sonography, a Complementary Examination to Alpha-fetoprotein Testing for Fetal Neural Tube Defects, *J Ultrasound Med*, 1985, 4; 307–10.

E. B. Hook and P. K. Cross, 'Interpretation of Recent Data Pertinent to Genetic Counselling for Down Syndrome: Maternal-age-spe-cific-rates, temporal trends, adjustments for paternal age, recur-rence risks, risks after other cytogenetic abnormalities, recur-rence risk after remarriage, in A. M. Willey, T. P. Carter, S. Kelly and I. H. Porter (eds), *Clinical Genetics: Problems in Diagnosis and Counseling*, Academic Press, New York, 1982, pp. 119–39.

E. B. Hook, P. K. Cross, L. Jackson, E. Pergament and B. Brambati, 'Maternal Age-specific Rates of 47, +21 and Other Cytogenetic Abnormalities Diagnosed in the First Trimester of Pregnancy in Chorionic Villus Biopsy Specimens: comparison with rates ex-pected from observations at amniocentesis', *Am J Hum Genet* 1988, 42, 797–807.

S. G. Ratcliffe and N. Paul, Prospective Studies on Children with Sex Chromosome Aneuploidy, Liss, New York 1986

## Chapter 6

B. F. Crandall, J. Howard, T. B. Lebherz et al, 'Follow-up of 2000 Second-Trimester Amniocenteses', *Obstet Gynecol* 1980, 56, 625–8.

L. Ch. de Crespigny, and H. P. Robinson, 'Amniocentesis: a com-parison of "Monitored" versus "Blind" needle insertion tech-nique, *Aust NZ J Obstet Gynaecol* 1986, 26, 124–8.

B. Elejalde, M. de Elejalde, J. M. Acunda et al, 'Prospective study of amniocentesis performed between weeks 9 and 16 of gestation', *Am J Med Genet* 1990, 35, 188–96.

Katayama K. P., Roesler M. R. 'Five Hundred Cases of Amniocentesis without bloody tap', *Obstet Gynecol* 1986, 68, 70–3.

W. F. O'Brien, 'Midtrimester Genetic Amniocentesis. A review of fetal risks', *J Reprod Med* 1984, 29, 59–63.

L. Pijpers, M. G. Jahoda, R. P. Vosters et al, 'Genetic Amniocentesis in twin pregnancies', *Br J Obstet Gynaecol* 1988, 95 323–326.

A. Tabor, J. Philip, M. Madsen et al, 'Randomised Controlled trial of genetic amniocentesis in 4606 low-risk women', *Lancet* 1986, 1, 1287–93.

M. Verjaal and N. J. Leschot, 'Risk of Amniocentesis and Laboratory Findings in a series of 1500 Prenatal Diagnoses', *Prenat Diagn* 1981, 1, 173–81.

R. A. Williamson, M. W. Varner, S. S. Grant, 'Reduction in Amniocentesis Risks Using a Real-time Needle Guide Procedure', *Obstet Gynecol* 1985, 65, 751–5.

## Chapter 7

A. Boogert, A. Mantingh and G. Visser, 'The Immediate Effects of Chorionic Villus Sampling on Fetal Movements', *Am J Obstet Gynecol*, 1987, 157, 137–9.

B. Brambati, A. Lanzani and L. Tului, 'Transabdominal and Transcervical Chorionic Villus Sampling. Efficiency and risk evaluation of 2411 cases', *Am J Med Genet* 1990, 35, 160–4.

B. Brambati, L. Tului, G. Simoni and M. Travi, 'Prenatal diagnosis at six weeks', *Lancet* 1988, 2, 397.

Canadian Collaborative CVS-Amniocentesis clinical trial group, 'Multicentre randomised clinical trial of chorion villus sampling and amniocentesis', *Lancet* 1989, 1, 1–6.

L. de Crespigny, H. Robinson and A. Ngu, 'Pain with amniocentesis and transabdominal CVS', *Aust NZ J Obstet Gynaecol* 1990, 30 308–9.

A. G. Hunter, H. Muggah, B. Ivey, D. M. Cox, 'Assessment of the Early Risks of Chorionic Villus Sampling', *Can Med Assoc J* 1986, 134, 753–6.

L. Jackson, 'CVS latest news', Division of medical genetics, Jefferson Medical College, Philadelphia, May 1990, No 28.

G. Monni, G. Olla and A. Cao, 'Patient's Choice between Transcervical and Transabdominal Chorionic Villus Sampling', *Lancet* 1988, 1, 1057.

G. C. Rhoads, L. G. Jackson, S. E. Schlesselman et al, 'The Safety and Efficacy of Chorionic Villus Sampling for Early Prenatal Diagnosis of Cytogenetic Abnormalities', N Engl J Med 1989, 320, 609–17.

G. Robinson, D. Garner, M. Olmsted et al, 'Anxiety Reduction after Chorionic Villus Sampling and Genetic Amniocentesis', *AMJ Obstet Gynecol* 1988, 159, 953–6.

H. P. Robinson, L. de Crespigny, A. Ngu et al, 'Transabdominal Chorionic Villus Sampling' — A safe and reliable procedure. In press.

J. Spencer and D. Cox, 'A Comparison of Chorionic Villi Sampling and Amniocentesis; acceptability of procedure and maternal attachment to pregnancy', *Obstet Gynecol* 1988, 72 714–17.

## Chapter 8

Keeley & Bean (eds), *Australian Attitudes*, Allen & Unwin, Sydney, 1988.

Tabor et al, ibid.

Spencer and Cox, ibid.

Robinson et al, ibid.

S. L. Clark and G. R. DeVore, 'Prenatal Diagnosis for Couples who Would Not Consider Abortion', *Obstet Gynecol* 1989, 73, 1035–7.

## Chapter 9

N. Wald, H. Cuckle, J. Densem et al, 'Maternal Serum Screening for Down's, syndrome in Early Pregnancy', *Br Med J* 1988, 297, 883–7.

S. C. Yeoh, I. L. Sargent, C. W. G. Redman and S. L. Thein, 'Detecting Fetal Cells in Maternal Circulation', *Lancet* 1989, 2, 869–70.

## Chapter 10

P. Boulot, F. Deschamps, G. Lefort et al, 'Pure Fetal Blood Samples Obtained by Cordocentesis; technical aspects of 322 cases', *Prenatal Diagnosis* 1990, 10, 93–100.

F. Daffos, M. Capella-Pavlowsky, F. Forestier, 'Fetal Blood Sampling During Pregnancy with Use of a Needle Guided by Ultrasound, a study of 606 consecutive cases', *Am J Obstet Gynecol* 1985, 153, 655–60.

M. J. Whittle, 'Cordocentesis', *Br J Obstet Gynaecol* 1989, 96, 262–4.

# INDEX

# The Crimson Cavalier